YEAR BOOK OF DERMATOLOGY – 2018

PSORIASIS

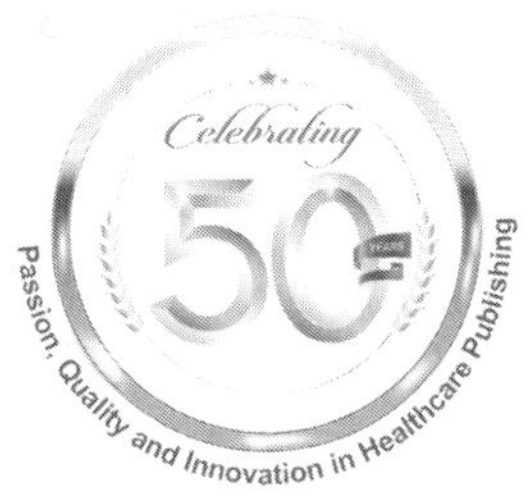

YEAR BOOK OF DERMATOLOGY – 2018

PSORIASIS

Editor

Jayakar Thomas MD DD MNAMS FRCP FRCPCH PhD DSc
Professor and Head
Department of Dermatology
Sree Balaji Medical College and Hospital
Chennai, Tamil Nadu, India

Foreword

Parimalam Kumar MD DD MNAMS FRCP

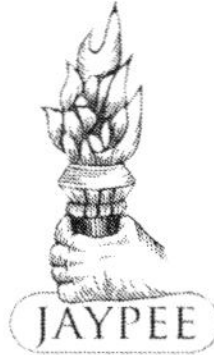

JAYPEE BROTHERS MEDICAL PUBLISHERS
The Health Sciences Publisher
New Delhi | London | Panama

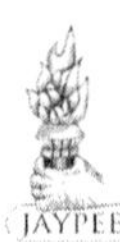

Jaypee Brothers Medical Publishers (P) Ltd

Headquarters

Jaypee Brothers Medical Publishers (P) Ltd
4838/24, Ansari Road, Daryaganj
New Delhi 110 002, India
Phone: +91-11-43574357
Fax: +91-11-43574314
Email: jaypee@jaypeebrothers.com

Overseas Offices

J.P. Medical Ltd
83 Victoria Street, London
SW1H 0HW (UK)
Phone: +44 20 3170 8910
Fax: +44 (0)20 3008 6180
Email: info@jpmedpub.com

Jaypee-Highlights Medical Publishers Inc
City of Knowledge, Bld. 235, 2nd Floor, Clayton
Panama City, Panama
Phone: +1 507-301-0496
Fax: +1 507-301-0499
Email: cservice@jphmedical.com

Jaypee Brothers Medical Publishers (P) Ltd
17/1-B Babar Road, Block-B, Shaymali
Mohammadpur, Dhaka-1207
Bangladesh
Mobile: +08801912003485
Email: jaypeedhaka@gmail.com

Jaypee Brothers Medical Publishers (P) Ltd
Bhotahity, Kathmandu, Nepal
Phone: +977-9741283608
Email: kathmandu@jaypeebrothers.com

Website: www.jaypeebrothers.com
Website: www.jaypeedigital.com

Inquiries for bulk sales may be solicited at: jaypee@jaypeebrothers.com

Year Book of Dermatology – 2018 *Psoriasis* / Jayakar Thomas

First Edition: **2019**

ISBN: 978-93-5270-593-1

Printed at Nutech Print Services, India

Dedicated to

The many dermatologists who provide care to their patients with psoriasis, to our committed teachers, and most of all to our beloved spouses for their care, love, affection, and support without which this humble piece of work would not have been a reality.

CONTRIBUTORS

Editor

Jayakar Thomas MD DD MNAMS FRCP FRCPCH PhD DSc
Professor and Head
Department of Dermatology
Sree Balaji Medical College and Hospital
Chennai, Tamil Nadu, India

Contributing Authors

Deepthi Ravi MD MRCP
Assistant Professor
Department of Dermatology
Sree Balaji Medical College and Hospital
Chennai, Tamil Nadu, India

Sobimeena RM MD
Senior Resident
Department of Dermatology
Sree Balaji Medical College and Hospital
Chennai, Tamil Nadu, India

Vignesh NR MD
Senior Resident
Department of Dermatology
Sree Balaji Medical College and Hospital
Chennai, Tamil Nadu, India

FOREWORD

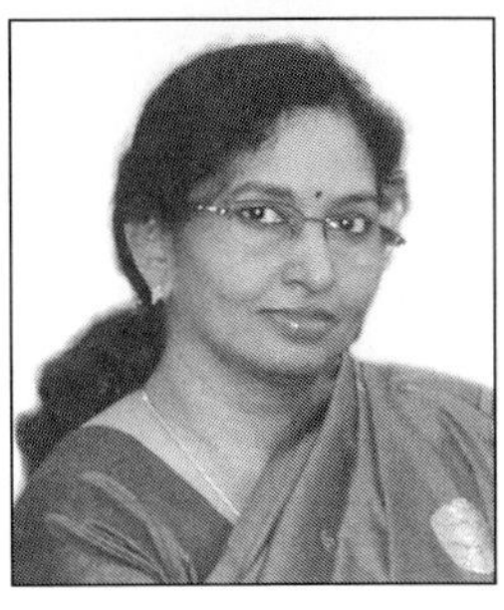

Parimalam Kumar MD DD MNAMS FRCP
Professor and Head
Department of Dermatology
Stanley Medical College,
Chennai, Tamil Nadu, India

It is indeed a privilege and pleasure to pen these lines of foreword for the title "Year Book of Dermatology – 2018 *Psoriasis*", edited by Professor Jayakar Thomas. I say this because I know him as a voracious reader, popular teacher, and a masterly orator, and also a great descriptive writer. I have been reading his several works—original articles, chapters in books, and also his other books. Above all, I have worked with him as co-editor in several titles.

The practice of medicine requires the acquisition of knowledge and skills, and the learning of attitudes and behaviors, apart from the manner in which it is disseminated. Professor Jayakar Thomas has exemplified this in this title "Year Book of Dermatology – 2018 *Psoriasis*".

"Year Book of Dermatology – 2018 *Psoriasis*" is a compilation of some of the recent literature pertaining to various aspects of psoriasis. The authors have skillfully written their analytical comments on the articles and the end of each one sees the key messages to the same. This makes easy and interesting reading.

Speaking volumes about the motivation driven by Professor Thomas is the effort put in by the young contributors. I congratulate the contributors Dr Deepthi Ravi, Dr Sobimeena RM, and Dr Vignesh NR for working in liaison with Professor Thomas.

It is my opinion that this book needs to be placed in the hands of all dermatologists.

I convey to Professor Jayakar Thomas and the contributors all my best wishes to more and more similar work towards academic excellence.

PREFACE

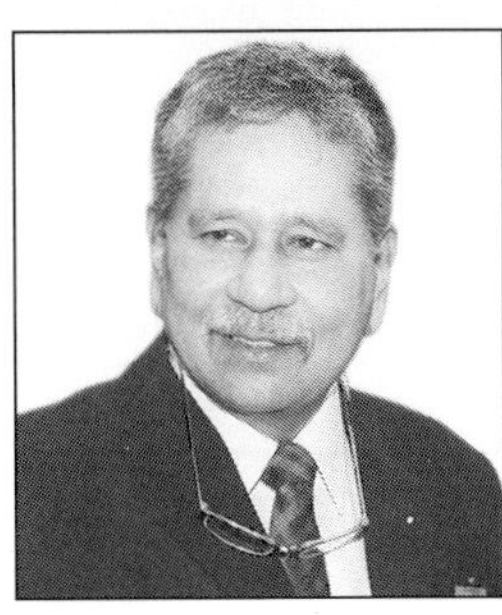

Jayakar Thomas MD DD MNAMS FRCP FRCPCH PhD DSc
Professor and Head
Department of Dermatology
Sree Balaji Medical College and Hospital
Chennai, Tamil Nadu, India

Psoriasis is the most common noncommunicable dermatologic disease seen in practice. Little wonder that bundles of papers are being published on psoriasis on a daily basis.

In this title "Year Book of Dermatology – 2018 *Psoriasis*", we have put in our best efforts to pick on some articles from recent literature and compile our views and comments on the same. We thank the original authors for their contribution.

We do hope that this book serves as a useful study guide to all our colleagues.

CONTENTS

ARTICLE 1

Apremilast in Psoriasis–A Prospective Real-world Study

Vujic I, Herman R. Sanlorenzo M, et al. Apremilast in psoriasis - A prospective real-world study. *J Eur Acad Dermatol Venereol. 2018;32(2):254-9.*

Abstract

Apremilast is an oral phosphodiesterase-4 inhibitor approved for the treatment of psoriasis. Various phase III trials have proved it to be safe and efficacious. This article is a prospective real-world study on the use and safety of apremilast in psoriasis and also to calculate the drug survival. About 48 patients were given apremilast and were evaluated every 4 weeks. The parameters evaluated were weight, height, age, joint involvement, PASI score, adverse effects and previous treatments. PASI 50, PASI 75 and PASI 90 were used to assess the efficacy of treatment.

COMMENT

This article is a prospective real-world study of the effect of apremilast in psoriasis patient. Apremilast is an oral phosphodiesterase-4 inhibitor used for psoriasis and psoriatic arthritis treatment.

A total of 48 patients were included in the study and the study was conducted over a period of 1 year 9 months.

The parameters studied were the drug survival (time from initiation to discontinuation of therapy) and the efficacy which was analyzed by means of PASI 50, PASI 75 and PASI 90 (Improvement in the psoriasis area severity index by 50, 75 and 90 points respectively).

The patients were followed up every 4 weeks and the parameters which were recorded in the proforma included the weight, height, age, family history, treatment history, presence of joint involvement, smoking status, PASI scores and the adverse effects if any (onset and duration).

The median drug survival was 12.5 weeks which can also be used as a measure of efficacy of the drug and compliance. PASI 50, PASI 75 and PASI 90 were achieved by eight, nine, and three patients respectively.

There was a negative impact of obesity on the PASI 50 response. Obese individuals have shown a less response to treatment in other studies as well and they also present with more severe disease.

Only 31 patients had adverse effects, the most common of which was diarrhea followed by headache and joint pain but none severe enough to stop treatment.

The trials done for apremilast in were ESTEEM and PALACE which showed significant greater results than in this real-world trial.

More long-term studies with a larger number of subjects are needed on apremilast to confirm these findings. Wide spread availability of apremilast with cost-effective rates in developing countries compared to developed countries will help in performing these studies.

Key Messages

- ***Even with the difference in the results between trial and real-world patients, apremilast has shown to be effective in the treatment of psoriasis with up to 40% patients reaching PASI 50 or higher***
- ***Body weight affects drug response with considerably less response being seen in obese individuals.***

ARTICLE 2

Comparative Effectiveness of Abatacept, Apremilast, Secukinumab and Ustekinumab Treatment of Psoriatic Arthritis: A Systematic Review and Network Meta-analysis

Kawalec P, Holko P, Moćko P, et al. Comparative effectiveness of abatacept, apremilast, secukinumab and ustekinumab treatment of psoriatic arthritis: A systematic review and network meta-analysis.
Rheumatol Int. 2018;38(2):189-201.

Abstract

The objective of this article was to find out the comparative efficacy and safety of biologic therapies especially non-anti TNF-α agents in the treatment of psoriatic arthritis.

A systematic review and meta-analysis was done according to PRISMA requirements by two investigators of several studies including randomized control trials. The criteria taken into consideration were ACR20, ACR50, PASI, PASI 75, safety outcomes and serious adverse effects. Secukinumab gave the best ACR20 endpoint in patients who were not treated with anti-TNF- α whereas secukinumab and apremilast had the highest benefit in patients previously treated with anti-TNF-α. Secukinumab was safest in terms of overall adverse effects, whereas ustekinumab had the lowest risk of severe adverse effects.

COMMENT

This article is a review and meta-analysis to compare the efficacy and safety of non-anti-tumor necrosis factor-α (TNF-α) novel biologic therapies in the treatment of psoriatic arthritis (PsA).

Traditionally treatment for PsA starts with disease-modifying antirheumatic drugs and non-steroidal anti-inflammatory drugs. If the patient does not respond or is intolerant to this, then tumor necrosis factor-α inhibitors (TNF-α I) such as etanercept, golimumab, infliximab and adalimumab are used. In patients who show primary or secondary non-responsiveness to TNF-α I, other biologics need to be given such as abatacept, secukinumab, ustekinumab, and small molecules such as apremilast.

Ustekinumab is a human immunoglobulin G1 which binds to the common p40 subunit which is present in both IL-23 and IL-12 and is involved in PsA pathogenesis. Secukinumab is a human immunoglobin-G1 monoclonal antibody which binds selectively and neutralizes IL-17A. Abatacept is a full human fusion protein which binds to CD86 and CD80 and thus inhibits T cell activation and decreases serum levels of inflammatory proteins and cytokines which are involved in PsA pathogenesis. Apremilast is oral phosphodiesterase 4 inhibitor that increases expression of anti-inflammatory mediators like IL-10 and decreases the expression of inflammatory cytokines.

Ustekinumab, apremilast, secukinumab and abatacept need to be used for a period of 28, 24, 16–24 and 24–26 weeks respectively and hence follow-ups in trials with similar duration were taken for the review.

The parameters studied were ACR20 (American College of Rheumatology 20% improvement) criteria, Psoriasis Area Severity Index (PASI) score, PASI 50, PASI 75 and PASI 90.

Eligible studies were identified by searching MEDLINE via Cochrane library, Embase and PubMed and a systematic review was done using the recommendations and methods from PRISMA extension statement for reporting of systematic reviews.

In anti-TNF-α naïve population, abatacept and secukinumab were better and in patients with anti-TNF-α-failure secukinumab and apremilast were better followed by ustekinumab when ACR20 was considered. Secukinumab 150 mg and ustekinumab were safest options considering severe adverse effects and withdrawals.

Key Messages

- ***Secukinumab in a dose of 150 mg and 300 mg had the highest ACR20 endpoint in overall population and anti-TNF-a-naive subpopulation.***
- ***In the anti-TNF-a-failure population, secukinumab 300 mg and apremilast 30 mg had the highest rank***
- ***Secukinumab in a dose of 300 mg was the safest when any adverse effects were considered and ustekinumab in a dose of 90 mg was safest when risk of severe adverse effects were considered.***

ARTICLE 3

Management of Common Side Effects of Apremilast

Langley A, Beecker J. Management of common side effects of apremilast.
J Cutan Med Surg. 2018;22(4):415-21.

Abstract

Apremilast is a new small molecule which inhibits phosphodiesterase 4 and thereby inhibits the production of pro-inflammatory cytokines and increases the synthesis of anti-inflammatory cytokines. Though this is portrayed as a safer drug, it is not free from side effects. The commonly reported side effects reported are nausea, diarrhea, headache and nasopharyngitis. Though these side effects are easily manageable, adequate counseling to the patient before starting the drug is necessary, as it may lead to non-adherence and discontinuation by the patient himself/herself. This article provides the clear management of the side effects noted with the approved dose of 30 mg BD dosing of apremilast.

COMMENT

Apremilast is indicated for the treatment of moderate-to-severe psoriasis in patients who could not tolerate other systemic agents or those in which phototherapy could not be given. This drug can also be given in psoriatic arthritis when the other classical disease-modifying antirheumatic drugs (DMARDs) fail to provide response. This drug acts by inhibiting phosphodiesterase 4, wherein the intracellular levels of cyclic adenosine monophosphate (cAMP) increase due to its decreased degradation and thereby the levels of pro-inflammatory cytokines like Tumor necrosis factor (TNF)-α, IL-17 and IL-23 are decreased. The drug is safe but has relatively mild side effects like nausea, vomiting, diarrhea and nasopharyngitis.

Various clinical trials have been conducted to determine the safety and efficacy of apremilast in the long-term treatment of psoriasis. The trials which have been conducted so far are the ESTEEM 1, ESTEEM 2, PALACE 1 and PALACE 2. These studies are the pioneers that lead the Food and Drug Administration (FDA) to approve the drug in 2014 for the said indication. Other trials for apremilast include the LIBERATE, phase 3 trial by Ohtsuki et al. and phase 2 trial by Papp et al. In this article the data from Ohtsuki et al. are presented which included the approved 30 mg twice daily dosing of apremilast. The clinical trial for psoriatic arthritis included the ACTIVE trial which presented the results of its phase 3b trial on 2016.

The incidences of the common side effects are presented in terms of exposure adjusted incidence rates (EAIR). In this article, the EAIR from all the studies except for ACTIVE will be provided.

The most frequently reported side effect of apremilast is diarrhea. Diarrhea is commonly seen during the first 2 weeks of treatment with apremilast and does not last longer than 1 month. The diarrhea is usually self-limiting and severe medications can be used to control it. The drugs commonly used are loperamide and bismuth subsalicylate. Treatment for diarrhea was given in 12% of patients in ESTEEM trials and 21% of patients in PALACE trials. The diarrhea caused by apremilast is mainly secretory in nature, the mechanism is due to inhibition of phosphodiesterase 4 enzyme which causes accumulation of cAMP in the enterocytes lining the gut mucosa which in turn activate the chloride channels. The activated chloride channels promote fluid secretion into the lumen diluting the luminal contents. However, the diarrhea caused by this mechanism does not last more than 2 weeks due to upregulation of other compensatory phosphodiesterases. The initial management for diarrhea includes adequate hydration, taking split meals and avoiding foods like dairy products and caffeine. Refractory diarrhea defined by three or more loose/liquid stools per day can be treated with fiber supplementation like psyllium husk powder. The drugs which can be used are bismuth subsalicylate and loperamide. If the problem persists even after treatment, opinion from medical gastroenterologist can be obtained and later adjustment of the dose or discontinuation can be done.

The second commonly reported side effect is nausea. The mechanism for nausea in these patients are due to increased trigger of chemoreceptor trigger zone and action on central neurokinin receptors. Management for nausea includes following general measures like adequate hydration, taking split meals, avoiding exercise and avoiding excessive water during meals. Drugs like diphenhydramine, ondansetron, amitriptyline and promethazine can be given if general measures fail.

The third common side effect in apremilast patients is headache. The mechanism of headache is not known. Initial measures like adequate sleep, adequate hydration and managing stress levels. Drugs like acetaminophen can be taken for initial management. Later non steroidal anti-inflammatory drugs (NSAIDs) can be given if the headache is severe.

The other side effect noted with apremilast is nasopharyngitis/upper respiratory tract infection. The general measures like hydration, sleep, avoiding nasal irritants and practicing hand hygiene are advised. Drugs like nasal decongestants and analgesics can be used.

Key Messages

- *Apremilast is a safe drug approved for moderate-to-severe psoriasis*
- *Side effects noted with this drug are nausea, diarrhea, headache and nasopharyngitis*
- *The above-mentioned side effects can be managed with general measures and if severe, with drugs*
- *If the side effects are very severe, discontinuation of the drug or dose alteration can be done.*

ARTICLE 4

Apremilast for the Treatment of Moderate-to-Severe Palmoplantar Psoriasis: Results from a Double-Blind, Placebo-Controlled, Randomized Study

Bissonnette R, Haydey R, Rosoph LA, et al. Apremilast for the treatment of moderate-to-severe palmoplantar psoriasis: Results from a double-blind, placebo-controlled, randomized study.
J Eur Acad Dermatol Venereol. 2018;32(3):403-10.

Abstract

Palmoplantar psoriasis has a significant effect on the quality of life of patients. Apremilast has been known to have significant benefit in palmoplantar psoriasis especially in combination with acitretin and/or phototherapy. The objective of this study was to evaluate the effect of treatment of moderate-to-severe palmoplantar psoriasis with apremilast on the work productivity and the quality of life of patients.

COMMENT

This was a randomized, double-blind, placebo-controlled study to assess the use of apremilast in the treatment of moderate-to-severe palmoplantar psoriasis. Apremilast is a phosphodiesterase 4 inhibitor used for the treatment of psoriasis and psoriatic arthritis.

In this study, 100 patients with moderate-to-severe palmoplantar psoriasis were studied. They were randomized into two groups. One group received apremilast in a dose of 30 mg twice a day and the second group received placebo. This was given for a period of 16 weeks. At the end of week 16, both groups received apremilast in a dose of 30 mg twice a day which was continued till week 32.

The endpoint studied was the ratio of patients achieving a PPPGA (Palmoplantar Psoriasis Physician Global Assessment) of 0 or 1 by the end of week 16.

No significant difference was seen in the proportion of patients achieving a PPPGA or 0/1 in the two groups by week 16 [($p = 0.1595$) <0.05]. At the end of 32 weeks of treatment a PPGA of 0/1 was achieved by 24% of the patients.

Even though there was no significant increase in proportion of patients achieving a PPGA of 0/1 in the apremilast group, there was a significant improvement in secondary end-points in the apremilast group.

There was greater proportion of achievement of PPPASI 75 (75% reduction in the palmoplantar psoriasis area severity index), in improvement of PPASI, reduction of activity impairment and improvement in Dermatology Life Quality Index (DLQI).

Further long-term studies are needed to confirm the findings in this study and to assess attainment of PPPGA of 0/1.

Key Message

- ***There is a significant improvement in the PPASI, reduction of activity impairment, improvement in quality of life and achievement of PPPASI 75 in patients with palmoplantar psoriasis as compared to placebo even though the difference proportion of patients achieving a PPGA of 0/1 was not statistically significant between the apremilast and placebo groups at week 16.***

ARTICLE 5

Long-term Safety and Tolerability of Apremilast in Patients with Psoriasis: Pooled Safety Analysis for ≥156 Weeks from 2 Phase 3, Randomized Controlled Trials (ESTEEM 1 and 2)

Crowley J, Thaçi D, Joly P, et al. Long-term safety and tolerability of apremilast in patients with psoriasis: Pooled safety analysis for ≥156 weeks from 2 phase 3, randomized, controlled trials (ESTEEM 1 and 2).
J Am Acad Dermatol. 2017;77(2):310-17.

Abstract

Various studies have been conducted regarding the safety and efficacy of apremilast but literature for long-term safety of apremilast is lacking. This randomized controlled trial was performed to analyze the long-term safety of oral apremilast, the finding reported for 0 to ≥156 weeks of exposure to the drug from the ESTEEM trial 1 and 2. The adverse events noted in the 0 to ≤52 weeks period were diarrhea, nausea, upper respiratory tract infection and headache. There was no new adverse event reported in the 0 to 156 week period. The serious adverse events like major cardiac events, malignancies and depression did not increase in comparison with the rates found during 0 to ≤52 week period. The limitations were high dropout rare. This study showed that apremilast has an acceptable safety profile and is generally well tolerated for 156 weeks.

COMMENT

Psoriasis is a chronic systemic inflammatory disease characterized by episodes of relapses and remissions. The current systemic agents used for the treatment of psoriasis cannot be used long-term considering the safety, tolerability and inconvenience for the patients due to periodic laboratory investigations and regular monitoring.

Apremilast is a phosphodiesterase 4 inhibitor, approved in the United States and Europe for the treatment of psoriasis and psoriatic arthritis. This randomized controlled trial (RCT) was conducted in various centers in the United States and Europe to demonstrate the efficacy and safety of apremilast for moderate to severe plaque psoriasis and psoriatic arthritis.

In this RCT, patients aged more than 18 years with moderate to severe plaque psoriasis who were candidates for systemic therapy were enrolled. At the end of the week 52 visit, patients were eligible to continue apremilast for up to 4 additional years.

Exposure-adjusted incidence rates (EAIRs) were used to assess major cardiac events, malignancies, and serious infections. Safety findings are reported for 0 to 156 weeks from ESTEEM 1 and 2. The 0 to 156 week period included 1184 patients, treated with 30 mg of apremilast taken twice daily.

During the first 52 weeks of drug exposure, the common side effects encountered in >5% of patients were diarrhea, nausea, upper respiratory tract infection, nasopharyngitis and headache. From 0 to ≥156 week period, the rates of serious adverse events (AEs) did not increase from the rates found during the 0 to ≤52 week period. The serious AEs in ≥2 patients in any exposure period included coronary artery disease, acute myocardial infarction, osteoarthritis and nephrolithiasis.

Rates of serious infections remained low with long-term apremilast exposure; there were no serious opportunistic infections or reactivations of TB infection and no significant changes in laboratory test/report values. Depression was extemporarily reported by few patients at week 16, but the incidence of depression did not increase with longer apremilast use.

The lack of impact of apremilast on blood cell counts, serious opportunistic infections, serious infections, and malignancies suggested that apremilast does not appear to have immunosuppressive effects such as those associated with cyclosporine or tofacitinib. The dropout rate in this study was high, but not because of safety concerns.

Apremilast is a safe and well tolerated drug which can be given long-term even in patients with comorbidities. The ease of administration, lack of laboratory monitoring and no specific organ toxicities makes it an enticing option for psoriasis patients.

Key Messages

- ***Apremilast is a safe and well tolerated drug which can be given long term even in patients with comorbidities***
- ***The ease of administration, lack of laboratory monitoring and no specific organ toxicities makes it an enticing option for psoriasis patients.***

ARTICLE 6

Secukinumab and Apremilast Combination Therapy for Recalcitrant Psoriasis

Hadi A, Lebwohl M. Secukinumab and apremilast combination therapy for recalcitrant psoriasis.
Journal of Psoriasis and Psoriatic Arthritis. 2017;2(2):59-60.

Abstract

Psoriasis is a chronic inflammatory disorder and affects the joints and the skin. It is associated with aberrant activity of Th1 and Th17 cells and is also associated with systemic inflammation. Many treatment options are available for psoriasis and combination treatment is also used. However a few cases are refractory to all modalities of treatment which indicates the need for newer innovative combination treatment for the management of refractory psoriasis and psoriatic arthritis. In this case report, a case of resistant plaque psoriasis was treated successfully with a combination of secukinumab and apremilast. This is the second reported case treated successfully with this combination.

COMMENT

This article is a case report of refractory psoriasis with psoriatic arthritis in a 61-year-old woman who treated with secukinumab and apremilast with significant improvement.

The patient has a 1-year history of psoriatic arthritis. She was initially started on adalimumab in a dose of 40 mg subcutaneously fortnightly. Subsequent to this she developed plaque psoriasis. This may be because of the development of paradoxical inflammatory disorders in patients treated with Tumor necrosis factor-α (TNF-α) inhibitors.

Subsequently the patient was treated with ustekinumab with no improvement which was followed by treatment with a combination of methotrexate and infliximab for a period of 10 months with not much improvement.

Secukinumab has already been proven to be effective in resistant cases of psoriasis in various studies. In this case, secukinumab produced a significant improvement in the psoriatic arthritis but only a modest improvement of the skin lesions. On introduction of apremilast, there was a significant improvement in both psoriasis and psoriatic arthritis. The patient was subsequently maintained on 300 mg of secukinumab monthly and 30 mg twice daily dose of apremilast with no adverse effects.

This is the second report of psoriasis patient resistant to other modalities of treatment being successfully treated with a combination of apremilast and secukinumab, the first being reported by Rothstein et al.

Apremilast is a phosphodiesterase4 inhibitor and has been shown to be effective in moderate-to-severe psoriasis. It has the benefits of being an oral therapy, not having the same risk of immunosuppression seen in biologics and not requiring any investigations for inception or monitoring of therapy. Apremilast has shown to be effective in combination with methotrexate, acitretin, cyclosporin, infliximab, adalimumab, ustekinumab and narrow-band ultraviolet B (NB-UVB).

Various combination therapies have been used in psoriasis which has proven to be effective in psoriasis refractory to monotherapy.

More case reports and studies are necessary to confirm the usefulness of secukinumab, apremilast combination in refractory psoriasis.

This combination may also prove to be expensive to the patient to continue on a long-term basis.

Key Messages

- ***Combination therapy of secukinumab and apremilast can be a promising treatment for the management of refractory psoriasis.***

ARTICLE 7

Apremilast: A Review in Psoriasis and Psoriatic Arthritis

Deeks ED. Apremilast: A review in psoriasis and psoriatic arthritis.
Drugs*. *2015;75(12):1393-403.

Abstract

Apremilast is an oral phosphodiesterase 4 inhibitor used for the treatment of adult psoriasis and psoriatic arthritis. Sustainable improvements up to 52 weeks in case of psoriasis and up to 104 weeks in case of psoriatic arthritis have been seen in ESTEEM and PALACE trials respectively. Both of these are phase III clinical trials. Improvement was seen within 16 weeks in both the trials.

COMMENT

This study is a review article on the use of apremilast in psoriasis and psoriatic arthritis (PsA). Apremilast is a small molecule administered orally and inhibits phosphodiesterase 4 (PDE-4). It acts intracellularly to modulate pro and anti-inflammatory mediators. PDE-4 inhibition increases cyclic adenosine monophosphate (cAMP) levels which down regulates inflammatory mediators such as Tumor necrosis factor-α (TNF-α), IL-23 and increases anti-inflammatory cytokines like Interleukin 10 (IL-10).

This article takes into consideration the two major clinical trial programs done for apremilast in psoriasis namely ESTEEM 1 and 2 (Efficacy and Safety Trial Evaluating the Effects of Apremilast in Psoriasis) and PALACE 1-3 (Efficacy and Safety Study of Apremilast to Treat Active Psoriatic Arthritis).

Apremilast showed significant improvement in the extent and severity of plaque psoriasis with improvement in the scalp, nail and palmoplantar lesions at 16 weeks with sustained benefits till 52 weeks as compared with placebo. Apremilast also showed significant improvement of PsA in patients even when treated with Disease-modifying antirheumatic drugs (DMARDs) in 16 weeks of treatment which was sustained till 104 weeks of treatment.

The most common early side effects were nausea and diarrhea which started in the first two weeks and resolved by 4 weeks of treatment. Upper respiratory tract infection and nasopharyngitis were seen in the later stages of treatment.

The review is based on only a few trials which were mainly conducted in western patients. A mention of a trial on Indian patients would also be helpful in guiding usage of this medication in the Indian subcontinent. Moreover, the ESTEEM trial had a high dropout rate of around 21% the reasons of which were not safety related. The cost of the medication may also prove to be a limiting factor in the usage of medication in India though the rates are less compared to biological agents.

Long-term tolerability and efficacy data would be useful especially since psoriasis is a chronic condition and medication is needed for a long period of time.

Key Messages

- ***The most common side effects in the initial stages of treatment with apremilast were nausea and diarrhoea and with continued treatment were upper respiratory tract infection and nasopharyngitis***
- ***Apremilast is a well-tolerated and effective drug in the treatment of psoriasis and psoriatic arthritis in adults with improvement in PsA being sustained for up to 104 weeks of treatment and improvement in skin lesions being sustained for up to 52 weeks of treatment.***

ARTICLE 8

Serum Squamous Cell Carcinoma Antigen in Psoriasis: A Potential Quantitative Biomarker for Disease Severity

Sun Z, Shi X, Wang Y, et al. Serum squamous cell carcinoma antigen in psoriasis: A potential quantitative biomarker for disease severity.

Dermatology. 2018;234(3-4):120-26.

Abstract

Serum squamous cell carcinoma antigen (SCCA) can be utilized to determine the association with disease severity and treatment in psoriasis patients. In this pilot study, 15 patients of psoriasis were treated with adalimumab after assessing psoriasis area and severity index (PASI) before and after treatment. The SCCA was detected using microparticle enzyme immunoassay. The SCCA levels were increased in patients with psoriasis and decreased levels were observed after treatment. Therefore, SCCA can serve as a useful quantitative biomarker for psoriasis disease activity.

COMMENT

Squamous cell carcinoma antigen (SCCA) is a member of serpin family, used in the diagnosis of squamous cell carcinoma. Localization of SCCA in psoriatic epidermis varies depending on its concentration in the patient's sera.

With low levels of the SCCA, weak and scattered staining could be noted in the granular layer. When the concentration is more, there is strong staining from the suprabasal to the granular layer and condensed staining around the plasma membranes and intercellular region was noted in the affected epidermis.

This study was done with the objective of using biomarkers like SCCA in association with disease severity and treatment response in psoriasis patients. In this study, 15 patients chosen were treated with adalimumab after calculating PASI score and body surface area (qBSA) before and after treatment.

SCCA was detected using microparticle enzyme immunoassay for both cases and controls. The serum SCCA level in psoriasis group was significantly higher than the control group. The levels of SCCA decreased after treatment and correlated well with PASI and qBSA.

SCCA contains two homologs, SCCA1 and SCCA2, which belong to the high molecular mass serine proteinase inhibitor superfamily, serpin. SCCA1 is very different from other serpins and inhibits papain-like cysteine proteinases, cathepsins K, L, and S. SCCA2 shows ordinary serpin-like properties and inhibits chymotrypsin-like serine proteinases, cathepsin G and mast cell chymase. SCCAs play a protective role against various proteinases in pathophysiologic events of psoriasis.

Upregulation of SCCA1 mRNA can be detected in the psoriatic skin when compared to the normal skin, whereas SCCA2 is not expressed in normal skin. SCCA2 is exclusively expressed in psoriatic skin. This suggests that SCCA1 is overexpressed in the psoriatic skin and SCCA2 is newly transcribed in psoriatic skin and is absent in normal skin.

Key Message

- ***Serum squamous cell carcinoma antigen might be a useful biomarker for detecting/testing psoriasis disease severity.***

ARTICLE 9

Long-term Real-life Safety Profile and Effectiveness of Fumaric Acid Esters in Psoriasis Patients: A Single-Centre, Retrospective, Observational Study

Dickel H, Bruckner T, Altmeyer P. Long-term real-life safety profile and effectiveness of fumaric acid esters in psoriasis patients: A single-centre, retrospective, observational study.
J Eur Acad Dermatol Venereol. 2018. doi:10.1111/jdv.15019.

Abstract

Fumaric acid esters (FAEs) are used in the treatment of moderate to severe psoriasis. The long-term safety and effectiveness of FAE either as a monotherapy or combination treatment is not known. Therefore, this monocentric retrospective, observational study was performed to assess the long-term safety and efficacy of FAE monotherapy or combination with other therapies. The most common side effect observed was in the gastrointestinal tract. Adverse events leading to treatment discontinuation were observed in 12.9% of patients. A median duration of 1 year was observed in all three treatment subcohorts ($p = 0.70$) from initiation of FAE treatment to a 50% response rate, where response was defined as achieving a cumulative static Physician's global assessment (PGA) score of 'light' and at least a 2-point reduction in baseline PGA. Therefore, this study reveals that FAE either as monotherapy or combination are safe and beneficial for long-term use.

COMMENT

Psoriasis is a chronic inflammatory autoimmune disease affecting the skin and the joints mediated by Th1, Th2 and Th22 cells. It is the most frequent immune mediated disease in humans. Patients with moderate to severe psoriasis generally require long-term or even lifelong systemic therapies.

Fumaric acid esters (FAEs) are recommended in European guidelines for the induction and long-term treatment of adults with moderate to severe psoriasis. Schweckendiek was the first to describe the use of fumaric acid for the treatment of psoriasis. Commercially available fumaric acid esters are a mixture of dimethyl fumarate and calcium and magnesium salts of monoethyl fumarate.

The current evidence suggests that monomethyl fumarate is the pharmacologically active compound with immunomodulatory properties particularly inhibiting Th17 and Th1 responses in psoriasis.

The objective of the study was to examine the long-term safety and effectiveness of FAEs as monotherapy and in combination with phototherapy or methotrexate in patients with psoriasis treated at a single center in Germany.

This was a monocentric, retrospective observational study with a follow-up period of 32.5 years. The study included 859 patients of which 626 received FAE monotherapy, 123 received FAEs with concomitant phototherapy and 110 received FAEs with methotrexate. All the patients additionally received other topical treatments for psoriasis.

The mean patient age group was 46.3 years. Approximately one-third of patients had family history of psoriasis and two-thirds were smokers. Approximately half of patients (49.0%) reported adverse events (566 total events), most of which involved the gastrointestinal tract. Usually, the gastrointestinal symptoms are mild to moderate and resolve with continued treatment.

In this study, the symptoms were rarely severe, requiring discontinuation of the treatment. The other common side effect was flushing of the skin, which is not serious and resolves with the administration of acetylsalicylic acid. Hematological disorders like lymphopenia and eosinophilia were the third most reported adverse effect. Although opportunistic infections are rare, 19 cases of progressive multifocal leukoencephalopathy had been identified in 19 cases taking FAE preparations.

Serious adverse events were reported in 2.3% of patients, but none seemed to have a causal relationship with any of the treatment regimens. Adverse events leading to treatment discontinuation were observed in 12.9% of patients. The mean duration of treatment required to achieve 50% response is 1 year when assessed with Physician's global assessment, whereas 50% response rate for achieving PASI 75 was achieved in 3 years with FAE monotherapy, 6.7 years in FAE + phototherapy subcohort and 8.1 years for FAE + methotrexate subcohort.

Though, novel fast acting and highly efficacious biologics have been introduced in the recent past, the authors opine that FAEs be used in the first-line of therapy for psoriasis as the therapy involves very less drug interactions and reasonable cost-benefit ratio in the long-term treatment.

Key Message

- ***Fumaric acid esters as monotherapy or in combination with phototherapy or methotrexate are safe and beneficial for long-term clinical use in psoriasis.***

ARTICLE 10

Association between Circulating 25-hydroxyvitamin D Levels and Psoriasis, and Correlation with Disease Severity: A Meta-analysis

Lee YH, Song GG. Association between circulating 25-hydroxyvitamin D levels and psoriasis, and correlation with disease severity: A meta-analysis.
Clin Exp Dermatol. 2018;43(5):529-35.

Abstract

Psoriasis is a chronic inflammatory disorder where 25-hydroxy vitamin D deficiency can contribute to the antiproliferative, anti-inflammatory and anti-angiogenic activities. This meta-analysis was performed to evaluate the relationship between circulating 25(OH)D levels and psoriasis, and its severity. In this analysis, 10 articles with 571 patients and 496 healthy controls (HCs) were included. The 25(OH)D level was significantly lower in the psoriasis group than in the HC group. Meta-analysis of the correlation coefficients revealed a small but statistically significant positive correlation between circulating 25(OH)D levels and PASI.

COMMENT

The biologically active form of vitamin D, 25-hydroxyvitamin D3 influences immune function as well as differentiation and growth of many cell types in addition to its central role in calcium and phosphate homeostasis. There is increasing evidence that vitamin D modulates responses of the innate and adaptive immune system resulting in inhibition of inflammation and enhancement of defense mechanisms. Many epidemiological studies have proclaimed the association of vitamin D and other chronic diseases like cardiovascular diseases, metabolic syndrome, malignancies and diseases of the brain.

The positive effects of ultraviolet B treatment in many chronic diseases and positive effects for inflammatory skin diseases following sun exposure, shows at least a partial role of vitamin D for the improvement of inflammatory changes. There is also evidence that a vitamin D deficit has an impact on mortality regardless of the risk of bone fracture. Since patients with severe psoriasis may die prematurely due to a significant increased risk for cardiovascular disease, a further evaluation of the role of vitamin D status might be of relevance for both prevention and treatment. The benefit of using vitamin D in the treatment of psoriasis is because of its action on vitamin D receptor in the keratinocytes leading to formation of responsive genes and finally helps in regulation of cell differentiation and reduces the proliferation.

The purpose of this study is to determine the association between vitamin D levels and the occurrence of psoriasis lesions and also to find out the association between the plasma levels of vitamin D and the austerity of the disease. The study revealed that the serum levels of vitamin D were decreased in psoriasis patients compared to the controls. The vitamin D levels could correlate with the disease severity which can be assessed by analyzing the Psoriasis Area Severity Index.

Despite increasing and convincing evidence for a significant role of vitamin D for central regulation of metabolism and the immune system, the preventive or therapeutic approach of vitamin D supplementation should always have a holistic view.

Key Messages

- ***Circulating 25(OH)D levels are lower in patients with psoriasis***
- ***Statistically significant negative correlation exists between 25(OH)D levels and psoriasis severity.***

ARTICLE 11

Maintenance of Skin Clearance with Ixekizumab Treatment of Psoriasis: Three-Year Results from the UNCOVER-3 Study

Leonardi C, Maari C, Philipp S, et al. Maintenance of skin clearance with ixekizumab treatment of psoriasis: Three-year results from the UNCOVER-3 Study.
J Am Acad Dermatol. 2018. pii: S0190-9622(18)30828-4.

Abstract

Ixekizumab (IXE) is a high-affinity monoclonal antibody which targets IL-17A used in moderate to severe psoriasis. This randomized controlled trial was conducted to evaluate efficacy and safety of IXE through 156 weeks from the UNCOVER-3 study in patients who received treatment up to

12 weeks with 160 mg initially followed by 80 mg every 2 weeks and 80 mg weekly thereafter. Patients were randomized to receive IXE every 2 weeks group and other group to receive every 4 weeks and other group with etanercept. At week 156, response rates were 80.5%, 66.0%, and 45.1% for PASI 75, 90 and 100 using mNRI method, respectively, and 97.2% and 86.2 for PASI 75 using as–observed and MI methods, respectively. This shows that IXE gives good response in clearance of skin and nail lesions.

COMMENT

Psoriasis is a chronic inflammatory disease mediated by aberrant immune responses and driven by self-perpetuating cytokine networks. Knowing the pathogenic cytokine network of psoriasis have led to the development of new treatments that provide greater efficacy in terms of complete skin clearance. Ixekizumab (IXE), a recombinant, high-affinity, humanized, IgG4-κ monoclonal antibody, selectively binds and neutralizes interleukin 17A (IL-17A), the proinflammatory and primary effector cytokine of type 17 helper T (Th17) cells. The UNCOVER-2 and UNCOVER-3 trials showed that after a 12-week induction period, IXE was superior to placebo and to twice-weekly etanercept for the treatment of moderate to severe psoriasis.

This study evaluates the efficacy and safety of IXE through 156 weeks from the UNCOVER-3 study in patients who received 160 mg of the drug at week 0, 80 mg every 2 weeks up to week 12 and 80 mg every 4 weeks thereafter. In the UNCOVER trial 3, after 3 months of receiving the above dosage of the drug, the patients entered a phase of maintenance during which the patients received 80 mg of IXE once a month up to approximately 13 months. In the UNCOVER trials 1 and 2, after the initial treatment with ixekizumab for 3 months, cases who had response to the drug were made to undergo randomization procedure into groups receiving the placebo treatment, another group where the drug was given at 80 mg dosage once a month, another group where they received drug at a dose of 80 mg every 3 months once and given up to 13 months. The treatment was considered to have reached the desired end point when there was attainment of Psoriasis Area Severity Index 75 at the end of third month.

This study was performed by randomizing the patients into four groups, the first were given IXE fortnightly, second were given IXE monthly once, third group received etanercept weekly twice and the last received placebo. All the groups were later given IXE monthly once and they entered the extension period.

The patients who received IXE experienced moniliasis compared to placebo the reason being that IXE blocks the interleukin 17 which plays a role in protection of mucosal surfaces from microbes. The study showed that there was risk for myocardial infarction when the levels of interleukin 17 decreases, but this cannot be generalized as an adverse effect and more studies are required to prove this.

Key Message

- *Ixekizumab sustained high responses with clearance of skin and nail lesions, with no new safety concerns through 3 years.*

ARTICLE 12

Psoriasis and the Risk of Diabetes: A Prospective Population-based Cohort Study

Wan MT, Shin DB, Hubbard RA, et al. Psoriasis and the risk of diabetes: A prospective population-based cohort study. *J Am Acad Dermatol. 2018;78(2):315-22.*

Abstract

This prospective population-based cohort study from United Kingdom was performed to determine the risk of type 2 DM in patients with psoriasis. This study included 8,124 patients with psoriasis and 76,559 adults without psoriasis and they were followed for a period of 4 years. There were 280 incident cases of DM in patients with psoriasis and 1,867 incident cases of diabetes in those without psoriasis. The limitation of this study is that a short-term follow-up of cases was followed.

COMMENT

Diabetes mellitus is a severe and growing public health problem worldwide. Psoriasis is a multifactorial, chronic immune-mediated inflammatory disorder of the skin, with a genetic component. Chronic inflammation contributes to both type 2 diabetes mellitus (T2D) and psoriasis. The association between the two diseases suggests a pathophysiologic link. In both diseases TH-1 and TH-17 cells are increased. These inflammatory mediators affect diverse processes, such as insulin resistance but also overeating, psychological stress and comorbidities, and release of inflammatory cytokines known to trigger psoriasis. A meta-analysis showed that the prevalence and incidence of T2D are increased among psoriasis patients. Moreover, systemic treatments for psoriasis might negatively affect cardiometabolic comorbidities.

This study was conducted to determine the risk for development of T2D in psoriasis patients comparing the adult population without psoriasis.

Metabolic control was worse in T2D patients with comorbid psoriasis. This may be probably due to reduced insulin sensitivity in psoriasis patients. A further reason might be the higher BMI in this patient group. Moreover, psoriasis T2D patients have to manage two diseases and thus the burden is increased. Therefore, diabetes self-care might be neglected despite requirement of more intensive medical care for T2D patients with psoriasis.

Key Message

- ***Clinicians may measure BSA affected by psoriasis to target diabetes prevention efforts for patients with psoriasis.***

ARTICLE 13

Psoriatic Patients with Chronic Viral Hepatitis do not have an Increased Risk of Liver Cirrhosis Despite Long-term Methotrexate Use: Real-world Data from a Nationwide Cohort Study in Taiwan

Tang KT, Chen YM, Chang SN, et al. Psoriatic patients with chronic viral hepatitis do not have an increased risk of liver cirrhosis despite long-term methotrexate use: Real-world data from a nationwide cohort study in Taiwan.
J Am Acad Dermatol. 2018; pii: S0190-9622(18)30659-5.

Abstract

Methotrexate (MTX) is the most commonly used drug in cases of moderate to severe psoriasis. This nationwide cohort study from Taiwan was done to determine the impact of long-term MTX use on the psoriatic patients with viral hepatitis associated cirrhosis. After a mean follow-up of more than 9 years since the diagnosis of chronic viral hepatitis, a total of 125 (5%) chronic hepatitis B (CHB) patients and 120 (11%) chronic hepatitis C (CHC) patients developed liver cirrhosis. This study shows that MTX use may not be associated with increased risk for liver cirrhosis in patients with chronic viral hepatitis.

COMMENT

Psoriasis (PsO) is a frequent inflammatory immunomediated disease affecting approximately 2% of the population. Patients with more extensive PsO (>10% of the body surface area) or psoriatic arthritis are in greater need of treatment. For these patients prolonged systemic therapies are often necessary. The therapeutic armamentarium available for the cure of PsO encompasses the conventional disease-modifying drugs (cDMARDs) and biological DMARDs (bDMARDs). The cDMARDS represent first-line of therapies in high need psoriatic patients, while bDMARDs are for those subjects in whom cDMARDs have either failed were not tolerated, or were contraindicated.

Psoriasis patients who are already infected with hepatitis B and hepatitis C viruses are challenging to receive parenteral drugs. Also the drugs which are administered can change the interaction between the host and the organism, and the underlying problem may become worse. Another problem is that the conventional DMARDs which are used have additional side effects which worsen the underlying condition.

This study was performed to investigate the use of methotrexate for long-term in patients of PsO with underlying hepatic cirrhosis which is viral induced. It was found that during follow-up from the initial diagnosis of viral hepatitis, approximately 5% of hepatitis B patients and 11% of hepatitis C patients had progressed to liver cirrhosis. The study recommends that all patients of psoriasis who are being planned for systemic therapy should be evaluated for serology of hepatitis B and C.

Key Message

- ***Long-term MTX use may not be associated with an increased risk of liver cirrhosis among psoriatic patients with chronic viral hepatitis.***

ARTICLE 14

Reporting of Outcomes in Randomized Controlled Trials on Nail Psoriasis: A Systematic Review

Busard CI, Nolte JYC, Pasch MC, et al. Reporting of outcomes in randomized controlled trials on nail psoriasis: A systematic review.
Br J Dermatol. 2018;178(3): 640-9.

Abstract

This systemic review was performed to identify the outcome instruments and corresponding outcome domains in nail psoriasis. The Nail Psoriasis Severity Index (NAPSI) was the most commonly used measure to assess clinical signs. Other outcome measures were measured using the nail area severity score, composite fingernail score, a Physician's global assessment, individual nail features. Variation in the type and reporting of nail psoriasis outcome instruments needs to be addressed in the process towards core outcomes set (COS) development.

COMMENT

Nail findings are often associated with skin lesions of psoriasis and the nature and number of pits helps to differentiate from other diseases and also to characterize the severity of disease. Greater number of pits also suggest the predisposition to develop psoriatic arthritis.

The presentation of nail psoriasis depends on the anatomical part which is involved in the disease process. The findings of nail involvement in nail psoriasis ranges from pits to splinter hemorrhages. The diagnosis is usually clinical but sometimes may require nail biopsy to differentiate from other conditions.

This study reviews the factors required for acquiring nail psoriasis. The aftermath of the disease process of nail psoriasis included the change in life quality index. The scoring system used to assess the disease process is Nail psoriasis Severity Index. Various studies evaluated the quality of life (QoL) affected by the disease process with only a few studies using a particular index for measurement.

Similar to psoriatic arthritis, nail psoriasis can also cause significant changes in the QoL. Many studies could not be conducted to evaluate the disease process of nail psoriasis due to its presentation, difficulty in treatment and inadequate response to treatment and irregular follow-up.

The treatment of nail psoriasis is challenging as it is usually resistant to therapy and requires adequate counseling of the patient regarding the disease process.

Key Messages

- ***Heterogeneity in the type and reporting of nail psoriasis outcome instruments needs to be addressed in the process towards COS development***
- ***Sufficient reporting of instrument characteristics should be encouraged***
- ***As nail psoriasis is generally assessed secondarily to psoriasis of the skin or joints, collaboration between different research groups in COS development is needed.***

ARTICLE 15

Risk of Cancer in Patients with Psoriasis on Biological Therapies: A Systematic Review

Peleva E, Exton L, Kelley K, et al. Risk of cancer in patients with psoriasis on biological therapies: A systematic review. ***Br J Dermatol. 2018;178(1):103-13.***

Abstract

The recent advances in the treatment of psoriasis are the biologicals, which though effective have profound effects on the immune system pathways and the immunosurveillance program. This systematic review was done to determine the risk of cancer in patients with psoriasis who are treated with biological therapy.

The incidence of non-melanoma skin cancer (NMSC) particularly squamous cell carcinoma was reported with TNF-α inhibitors (TNFi). There was no evidence for the increased of incidence other solid organ malignancies.

COMMENT

In the recent years, the use of biological drugs is increased for various indications ranging from psoriasis to pemphigus vulgaris. The biological agents though effective cause significant changes in the immune mechanisms of the body like cytokine production and causation of malignancies.

The side effects due to short-term use of biologicals is known but the risks in long-term use is not known. The biological drugs have been used for almost a decade and hence studies regarding the long-term side effects like malignancies due to biologicals can be performed.

This study was conducted to evaluate the risk of acquiring malignancies in patients of psoriasis who are treated with biological agents and follow-up period of 24 weeks minimum was fixed.

The study found that the incidence of squamous cell carcinoma was found to be high in patients receiving TNFi. The incidence of other solid organ malignancies was found to be minimum.

The results of this study cannot be applied to the entire population as the data included in this study comes from a particular geographic location, and there is difference in inherent susceptibility to cancers, in that particular location: these are the drawbacks and the latency period during which the malignancy develops in not analyzed in the studies included.

Key Messages

- ***Studies show an increased risk of NMSCs, especially SCC, for patients with psoriasis receiving the TNFi therapies etanercept and adalimumab compared with the general US population***
- ***The evidence to date suggests that there is no increased risk of cancers other than NMSC***
- ***Continued need for pharmacovigilance is required.***

ARTICLE 16

Safety of Adalimumab Dosed Every Week and Every Other Week: Focus on Patients with Hidradenitis Suppurativa or Psoriasis

Ryan C, Sobell JM, Leonardi CL, et al. Safety of adalimumab dosed every week and every other week: Focus on patients with hidradenitis suppurativa or psoriasis.
Am J Clin Dermatol. 2018;19(3):437-47.

Abstract

Adalimumab is a TNF-α inhibitor drug which is approved for use in psoriasis and hidradenitis suppurativa (HS). This placebo controlled, open label study was performed to examine the safety of administration of adalimumab every other week (EOW) or every week (EW) in the treatment of psoriasis and HS. The study revealed that there was no concerns regarding the safety whether the drug is administered EW or EOW.

COMMENT

Hidradenitis suppurativa (HS) is a disorder of the apocrine gland characterized by the recurrent lesions like abscesses, nodules, and scarring in the areas where the apocrine gland is maximum namely the axillary and groin regions. In patients with HS there is increased amount of TNF-α detected in the blood and sweat.

Adalimumab is a TNF-α inhibitor, a monoclonal antibody approved by the FDA for the management of severe HS and chronic plaque psoriasis. The dosage regimen of adalimumab in the management of patients with HS is by starting with a dose of 160 mg ensued by administering 80 mg dose 2 weeks, later the drug is given by

40 mg doses every week (EW). The dosage regimen of adalimumab in psoriasis patients is different; the regimen followed is starting dose of 80 mg ensued by 40 mg doses given every other week (EOW).

This study was performed to determine the regimen of adalimumab given either EW or EOW. The safety of adalimumab with the above mentioned dosing and regimen was studied from studies on HS, psoriasis, inflammatory bowel disease and rheumatoid arthritis.

It was observed that there was no increased risk for adverse effects when the drug was given EW. There was no significant difference observed between the above mentioned dosing schedules in cases of psoriasis and HS. The similar results were seen in other conditions like Crohn's disease, ulcerative colitis, and rheumatoid arthritis.

The above findings cannot be generalised to the whole population as there may be differences between the population like concomitant medication intake and other comorbidities. Statistical tests for safety data was not performed in this study.

Key Messages

- *It was observed that there was no increased risk for adverse effects when the drug was given every week*
- *There was no significant difference observed between the above mentioned dosing schedules in cases of psoriasis and HS.*

ARTICLE 17

Secukinumab Treatment of Moderate to Severe Plaque Psoriasis in Routine Clinical Care: Real-life Data of Prior and Concomitant Use of Psoriasis Treatments from the PROSPECT Study

Körber A, Thaçi D, von Kiedrowski R, et al. Secukinumab treatment of moderate to severe plaque psoriasis in routine clinical care: Real-life data of prior and concomitant use of psoriasis treatments from the PROSPECT study.
J Eur Acad Dermatol Venereol. 2018;32(3):411-9.

Abstract

Secukinumab is a fully human monoclonal antibody which targets IL-17 and various studies have proved its efficacy and safety in moderate to severe psoriasis. The literature regarding the duration of treatment with this agent as well as usage of concomitant pharmacologically active substances which will affect the safety and efficacy, and safety of secukiniumab is also unknown. This PROSPECT study was performed to assess the above mentioned factors. The results showed that the subjects included in this study had severe disease and the usage of other agents depended upon disease severity and the duration of treatment with secukinumab banked on prior treatment.

COMMENT

Secukinumab is a fully humanized anti-interleukin 17A monoclonal antibody with demonstrated efficacy in moderate to severe plaque psoriasis. Initially before administering secukinumab as per study protocols, previous treatments taken for psoriasis have to be stopped for a certain defined minimal length and concurrent psoriasis medication was prohibited. Therefore data regarding concomitant use, effectiveness and safety of other treatment for psoriasis with secukinumab is lacking.

To overcome the above mentioned short-coming, the PROSPECT study was designed to assess prior and concomitant use of psoriasis treatments in subjects receiving secukinumab. PROSPECT was an ongoing 24 week cohort study. Patients included in this study were those who had severe disease and who were willing for treatment with secukinumab.

Males were the dominant sex in this study with an average age group of 48 years. The PASI was recorded at the beginning of the treatment which had a mean of 18.

Before the subjects were included i.e., 1 year before, the subjects had received topical, systemic, or biologic treatments and 22% of subjects did not receive any treatment. Adverse effects leading to discontinuation of treatment was seen more with conventional systemic agents rather than biologicals.

Key Message

- ***The results showed that the subjects included in this study had severe disease and the usage of other agents depended upon disease severity and the duration of treatment with secukinumab banked on prior treatment.***

ARTICLE 18

Serum Levels of Psoriasin (S100A7) and Koebnerisin (S100A15) as Potential Markers of Atherosclerosis in Patients with Psoriasis

Awad SM, Attallah DA, Salama RH, et al. Serum levels of psoriasin (S100A7) and koebnerisin (S100A15) as potential markers of atherosclerosis in patients with psoriasis.
Clin Exp Dermatol. 2018;43(3):262-7.

Abstract

The proinflammatory cytokines which are upregulated in psoriasis are psoriasin and koebnerisin. This study was conducted to evaluate the role of psoriasin and koebnerisin in the subclinical atherosclerosis in psoriasis patients. Psoriasis patients with subclinical atherosclerosis had higher serum levels of koebnerisin compared with patients without subclinical atherosclerosis, which was not observed for psoriasin. This study shows that koebnerisin can be a useful marker for subclinical atherosclerosis.

COMMENT

Psoriasis is a systemic immune-mediated chronic inflammatory disease. In the skin, the antimicrobial proteins koebnerisin (S100A15) and psoriasin (S100A7) are overexpressed in the epidermis of psoriatic lesions and mediate inflammation as chemoattractant for immune cells. Their role for systemic inflammation in circulating leukocytes is unknown.

This study evaluates the role of serum psoriasin and koebnerisin as possible markers for subclinical atherosclerosis in psoriasis patients. In this study, the serum levels of psoriasin and koebnerisin were measured with ELISA in 45 patients and 45 controls. The intima-media thickness (IMT) of the right and left common carotid arteries was measured to detect the presence of subclinical atherosclerosis.

Compared with Healthy controls (HCs) patients with psoriasis had significantly higher levels of psoriasin and koebnerisin and significantly higher IMT values. A positive correlation was observed between IMT and Psoriasis Area and Severity Index (PASI) serum psoriasin and serum koebnerisin. Patients with psoriasis with subclinical atherosclerosis had higher serum levels of koebnerisin compared with patients without subclinical atherosclerosis, which was not observed for psoriasin.

Key Messages

- *Serum psoriasin and koebnerisin correlate with IMT, underlining their value as a potential link between psoriasis and atherosclerosis*
- *Koebnerisin seems to be a useful marker of subclinical atherosclerosis in patients with psoriasis.*

ARTICLE 19

Simulating the Life Course of Psoriasis Patients: The Interplay between Therapy Intervention and Marital Status

Linder M, Frigessi A, Piaserico S, et al. Simulating the life course of psoriasis patients: The interplay between therapy intervention and marital status.
J Eur Acad Dermatol Venereol. 2018;32:62-7.

Abstract

Psoriasis is a chronic disease with primary involvement of the skin and associated with multiple comorbidities like metabolic syndrome and cardiovascular involvement. In addition patients experience psychological problems like depression, anxiety, job loss and marital problems. This study was performed to evaluate the role of psychosocial factors and the clinical course of psoriasis. As increasing the number of variables leads to an exponential increase of the model's state space, switching to micro modeling (representing each individual separately) may be necessary.

COMMENT

Psoriasis primarily affects the skin with many comorbid conditions like depression and cardiovascular conditions associated with it. Psoriasis is associated with psychosocial problems like job loss, social isolation and partnership problems. Also the disease course runs an inverse relationship with the psychosocial problems.

This study was performed to determine the interaction of psychosocial and clinical parameters over the life of patients with psoriasis. In this study parameters like whether the patient is single or married, single and having a psoriasis flare, single and cured, coupled and healthy, coupled and having a psoriasis flare, coupled and cured, and dead were included. The data were taken from the Norwegian population register for the healthy population and from epidemiological research articles.

This study shows the effect of treatment intervention on the chances of living with a partner and also among the other mentioned states which are included.

Key Messages

- ***Complex models, comprising more variables are needed for more realistic simulations for the interactions studied***
- ***As increasing the number of variables leads to an exponential increase of the model's state space, switching to micro modeling may be necessary.***

ARTICLE 20

Smoking Paradox in the Development of Psoriatic Arthritis among Patients with Psoriasis: A Population-based Study

Nguyen UDT, Zhang Y, Lu N, et al. Smoking paradox in the development of psoriatic arthritis among patients with psoriasis: A population-based study.
Ann Rheum Dis. 2018;77(1):119-23.

Abstract

Literature has shown that smoking is associated with increased risk for psoriatic arthritis (PsA) but not in patients with psoriasis. This study was performed to analyze the association between smoking and development of PsA and also among patients with psoriasis. This shows that smoking was positively associated with PsA risk in the general population, but negatively associated among patients with psoriasis.

COMMENT

Psoriatic arthritis (PsA) is an inflammatory joint condition affecting an estimated 520,000 individuals in the US population. The unfavorable cutaneous and joint effects of smoking have been suggested from past studies due to the impact on the immune system and induction of oxidative stress. However, only sparse evidence regarding the association between smoking and PsA has been reported. This study was conducted to clarify the possible mechanisms behind the paradox.

It was found that in this study that smoking was associated with an increased risk of PsA in the general population, but with a less risk among patients with psoriasis. Mediation analysis revealed that the effect of smoking on the risk of PsA was interposed almost entirely through its effect on psoriasis.

Smoking induces oxidative stress and reduces antioxidant levels, leading to an imbalance of oxidants and antioxidants. The nicotinic cholinergic receptors in keratinocytes can be activated by smoking, subsequently stimulating calcium influx and accelerating cell differentiation. More importantly, smoking can adversely alter the immunological and inflammatory processes, and elevated levels of autoantibodies have been detected among smokers.

Key Message

- ***Smoking was positively associated with PsA risk in the general population, but negatively associated among patients with psoriasis.***

ARTICLE 21

Stricturing and Fistulizing Crohn's Disease is Associated with Anti-tumor Necrosis Factor-induced Psoriasis in Patients with Inflammatory Bowel Disease

Weizman AV, Sharma R, Afzal NM, et al. Stricturing and fistulizing Crohn's disease is associated with anti-tumor necrosis factor-induced psoriasis in patients with inflammatory bowel disease.
Dig Dis Sci. 2018. doi: 10.1007/s10620-018-5096-2.

Abstract

Studies have shown that the patients who are being treated with TNF-α inhibitors have paradoxical development of psoriasis. This study was performed to determine the prevalence and clinical characteristics of anti-TNF-associated psoriasis in a large cohort of inflammatory bowel disease patients. In a total of 676 patients who were treated with TNF-α inhibitors, the psoriasis incidence was found to be 10.7%. The time required for the development of psoriasis from the start of the therapy is approximately 569 days, with earlier onset being reported in patients with adalimumab rather than infliximab.

COMMENT

Inflammatory bowel disease (IBD) is a group of inflammatory disorders which include Crohn's disease (CD), ulcerative colitis (UC) and other unclassified. The cytokine which is implicated in the pathogenesis of the above mentioned disorders is tumor necrosis factor-α.

Patients who are administered TNF-α for the above conditions develop psoriasis as an enigmatic side effect, the causes of which is still unknown.

This study was conducted to determine the clinical characteristics of the development of psoriasis in IBD patients who are treated with TNF-inhibitor. This study included data from the hospital registry of tertiary care hospitals.

The patients who developed psoriasis during treatment were followed retrospectively to determine the dermatologic features.

Among 676 patients treated with anti-TNF, the incidence of psoriasis was 11%. The predisposing factors for developing psoriasis were females, stricturing or fistulizing Crohn's disease and upper Gastrointestinal (GI) Crohn's disease. The time required for the development of psoriasis from the initiation of the treatment was 1.5 years. Plaque psoriasis was the most common type of psoriatic lesion. Topical corticosteroids were the most common treatment for psoriasis.

Key Messages

- ***A high incidence of anti-TNF-associated psoriasis was associated with female gender, foregut disease location, and fistulizing and stricturing disease behaviour***
- ***More prospective studies and genetic analyses evaluating possible pathophysiologic underpinnings of this problem are needed.***

ARTICLE 22

Studying the Effect of Systemic and Biological Drugs on Intima-Media Thickness in Patients Suffering from Moderate and Severe Psoriasis

Martinez-Lopez A, Blasco-Morente G, Perez-Lopez I, et al. Studying the effect of systemic and biological drugs on intima-media thickness in patients suffering from moderate and severe psoriasis.
J Eur Acad Dermatol Venereol. 2018;32(9):1492-8.

Abstract

It is well known that the psoriasis has a link to a number of cardiovascular risk factors, hypertension and atherosclerosis. The carotid intima-media thickness (IMT) can be considered a marker for development of atherosclerosis. This study was performed to assess the effect of systemic and biological drugs which are used in psoriasis and changes observed in the carotid IMT with the therapy. The study has shown that treatment with biological drugs and methotrexate decreased the IMT levels. The study also showed that there is a decrease in glycemia and insulin levels in patients who are treated with tumor necrosis factor-α (TNF-α) inhibitors and ustekinumab.

COMMENT

The inflammatory events found in psoriasis pathogenesis are found to be similar in atherosclerosis. The increased carotid intima-media thickness (IMT) can serve as a marker of generalized arteriosclerosis.

This study was conducted to determine the effect of systemic chemotherapeutic agents and biological drugs on psoriatic patients' carotid IMT. In this study, a total of 53 patients requiring systemic therapy were included and sonogram of carotid IMT was performed before introducing the treatment. Also, follow-up scanning of carotid IMT was performed.

It was found in this study that the IMT of the patients with psoriasis treated with biological drugs tended to decrease with no statistical difference. Patients who were administered methotrexate and anti-IL-12/23 had a decrease in their IMT levels. A decline in sugar and insulin levels were noted in patients treated with tumor necrosis factor-α (TNF-α) inhibitors.

Many studies have shown results that the treatment of psoriasis with biologicals show improvement in the cardiovascular status and reduction of markers of atherosclerosis. The onset of this beneficial effect of these drugs is approximately 2 months after treatment initiation.

Key Messages

- *Carotid IMT may benefit from treatment with biological drugs, particularly anti-IL-12/23 and methotrexate in patients suffering from moderate and severe psoriasis*
- *Larger longitudinal studies should be performed to fully confirm these results.*

ARTICLE 23

Systemic Immune Mechanisms in Atopic Dermatitis and Psoriasis with Implications for Treatment

Guttman-Yassky E, Krueger JG, Lebwohl MG. Systemic immune mechanisms in atopic dermatitis and psoriasis with implications for treatment.
Exp Dermatol. 2018;27:409-17.

Abstract

Atopic dermatitis (AD) and psoriasis are chronic inflammatory disease that are characterized by erythematous, thickened epidermal lesions that vary in intensity and affected body surface area. Studies have shown that the pathogenesis of psoriasis involves Th1 pathway with Th17 cells are the main players in the pathogenesis of this disorder whereas the Th2 mediated immunity plays a role in the pathogenesis of AD. The Th17/IL-23 pathway also has an important role in psoriasis. The role of systemic inflammation in AD and psoriasis is supported by the occurrence of non-cutaneous comorbidities that affect patients, most of which intensify morbidity and disability associated with lesional skin. The success of agents like biologicals which are used in psoriasis drives a new approach in the treatment of moderate-to-severe AD.

COMMENT

Psoriasis and atopic dermatitis (AD) are associated with comorbid conditions that impair the quality of life. Recent studies link the inflammation related comorbidities between atopic dermatitis and psoriasis.

As with atopic march, psoriasis has been conceptualized with psoriatic march which denotes a characteristic progression of insulin resistance, endothelial dysfunction, atherosclerosis and cardiovascular events that has been observed in patients with moderate-to-severe psoriasis.

Atopic dermatitis is also linked to metabolic and cardiovascular diseases. Systolic and diastolic blood pressures are significantly increased in adolescents affected by moderate-to-severe AD. Atopic dermatitis is associated with increased risk of lymphoma tumors in the esophagus, lung and brain.

Patients with AD tend to be more susceptible to microbial infections at lesional sites, possibly because of reduced levels of IL-17-induced adenosine monophosphates (AMPs). In contrast to patients with AD, patients with psoriasis tend to have decreased susceptibility to cutaneous infections because of increased levels of AMPs.

Anxiety, suicidal ideation and depression are disproportionately increased in patients with AD and psoriasis. Adolescents with AD are at increased risk of development of attention deficit hyperactivity disorder.

These insights have led to novel therapeutics which aimed at addressing psoriasis by targeting tumor necrosis factor-α and Th17-related cytokine pathways. The success of these agents in psoriasis management is driving new therapeutic approaches for moderate-to-severe AD, including agents targeting the Th2 and Th17/Th22 cytokine pathways.

Key Messages

- ***Both atopic dermatitis (AD) and psoriasis are tightly linked with serious comorbidities***
- ***Topical agents addressing barrier function and local inflammation may not be sufficient to treat patients with moderate-to-severe AD***
- ***Continued exploration of the systemic mechanisms of AD will suggest new approaches to AD treatment and may modify existing psoriasis strategies.***

ARTICLE 24

The Akkermansia-muciniphila is a gut Microbiota Signature in Psoriasis

Tan L, Zhao S, Zhu W, et al. The Akkermansia-muciniphila is a gut microbiota signature in psoriasis. ***Exp Dermatol. 2018;27:144-9.***

Abstract

Psoriasis is a chronic immune mediated inflammatory skin disease in which the Th17 cells which produce IL-17, IL-22 and IL-23 plays a role in the pathogenesis of the disease. Recent studies have shown that gut microbiota plays a crucial role in host homoeostasis and immune response, particular in Th17 cells, but the role of the gut microbiota in psoriasis remains unclear. This study was performed to find out the association between gut microbiota and psoriasis using 16S rDNA sequencing. The results of this study is that Akkermansia-muciniphila has a main role in the pathogenesis of psoriasis, inflammatory bowel disease and obesity.

COMMENT

The etiology of psoriasis can be considered as polygenic in which in addition to genetic factors, environmental factors can play a role in the disease causation. The normal microflora of the skin plays an important role in maintaining the barrier function wherein it prevents the pathological organisms from entering the body. The role of microflora of the skin in the disease causation is established in disorders like psoriasis, atopic dermatitis and acne.

The alteration in the constitution of the skin microflora can mediate diseases of the immune origin. The pathogenesis of inflammatory bowel disease can also be correlated with changes in the cutaneous microflora causing changes in the immune system of the mucosa.

Literature regarding the role played by the cutaneous microflora and the Th17 immune response is available but their role in psoriasis pathogenesis is an enigma. This study was conducted to determine the role of microflora of the gut in the pathogenesis of psoriaisis.

This study identified that that Akkermansia-muciniphila, microbe found in the gut, to be decreased in psoriasis patients. Akkermansia-muciniphila can be considered as a marker of good health status and may play a role in the disease process of psoriasis and obesity.

The findings of this study reveal that in psoriasis patients there is a marked alteration in the microflora of the gut providing a new angle to approach the pathogenic process of psoriasis.

Key Messages

- *Akkermansia-muciniphila was significantly reduced in patients with psoriasis*
- *Akkermansia-muciniphila, which is an indicator of health status, may be a key node for psoriasis as well as IBD and obesity.*

ARTICLE 25

Topical Corticosteroid Concerns among Parents of Children with Psoriasis Versus Atopic Dermatitis: A French Multicentre Cross-sectional Study

Moawad S, Mahé E, Aubert-Wastiaux H, et al. Topical corticosteroid concerns among parents of children with psoriasis versus atopic dermatitis: A french multicentre cross-sectional study.
Am J Clin Dermatol. 2018;19:261-5.

Abstract

Topical therapies are the first-line of treatment in any disorder which involves less body surface area. In chronic inflammatory disorder like psoriasis and atopic dermatitis (AD) the gold standard treatment is topical corticosteroids. The fear of using topical steroids is well known among parents of children with AD, but not in psoriasis. TOPICOP is a helpful and easy-to-use tool for the evaluation of topical corticosteroid concerns (TCCs). It may help clinicians improve adherence to treatment and correct misconceptions. This cross-sectional multicentre study was performed to compare the TCC of parents of children with psoriasis or AD using the TOPICOP scale and a visual analog scale (VAS). The study shows that the TCC for both psoriasis and AD are the same.

COMMENT

Psoriasis and atopic dermatitis are chronic inflammatory disorders for which the gold standard treatment is topical steroids. These topical steroids can be used only when the disease is limited. If the disease is extensive, in psoriasis immunosuppressants like methotrexate, cyclosporine and other drugs are given, whereas in atopic dermatitis cyclosporine, azathioprine can be given.

Topical corticosteroids help in rapid resolution of the lesions, after which other steroid sparing agents like tacrolimus can be given in AD and vitamin D analogues and other drugs can be given in psoriasis. The fear of use of topical steroids in the treatment of AD is known but the same in psoriasis is not known.

TOPICOP is a useful and easy tool for studying the topical corticosteroid concerns (TCCs). It may help clinicians as well as patients/guardians to improve adherence to the treatment and correct misconceptions.

The aim of the study was to compare the TCC of parents of children with psoriasis or AD. This study can be considered new as the data regarding TCC concerns for psoriasis in pediatric population is very less.

The TOPICOP scale established for patients with AD has 12 questions to assess patients' worries and beliefs about topical corticosteroids. The parents were asked to fill up a standard questionnaire and also the visual analog scale (VAS) was completed.

Higher mean TOPICOP score was observed to be high if the mother answered. The TOPICOP score was high for AD patients when they were seen as outpatients and in psoriasis group; it was higher during the first visit. The results of this study show that the TCC for both psoriasis and AD are the same. This problem can be overcome by proper counseling of the parent regarding the appropriate use of steroids for a shorter period for the rapid control of the disease and use of other agents for maintenance.

Key Messages

- *TOPICOP is a helpful and easy-to-use tool for the evaluation of topical corticosteroid concerns (TCCs)*
- *The study shows that the TCC for both psoriasis and atopic dermatitis are the same.*

ARTICLE 26

Fumaric Acid Esters in Combination with a 6-week Course of Narrowband Ultraviolet B Provides an Accelerated Response Compared with Fumaric Acid Esters Monotherapy in Patients with Moderate-to-Severe Plaque Psoriasis: A Randomized Prospective Clinical Study

Tzaneva S, Geroldinger A, Trattner H, et al. Fumaric acid esters in combination with a 6-week course of narrowband ultraviolet B provides an accelerated response compared with fumaric acid esters monotherapy in patients with moderate-to-severe plaque psoriasis: A randomized prospective clinical study.
Br J Dermatol. 2018;178:682-8.

Abstract

Fumaric acid esters (FAEs) are a safer alternative to other systemic therapies used in psoriasis but these drugs have a slow onset of action. To overcome this disadvantage, the drug can be combined with other treatment modalities like narrowband ultraviolet B therapy (NB-UVB). This randomized assessor masked trial was performed to assess the synergistic effect of 6-week course of NB-UVB in addition to FAE in adults with moderate-to-severe plaque psoriasis. The results of this study are the mean reduction in PASI after 6 weeks was significantly greater with the combination treatment than with FAE monotherapy. This shows that adding a 6 week course of NB-UVB to FAE therapy could bring down the duration of treatment of psoriasis and also the quality of life.

COMMENT

Psoriasis is a chronic recurring inflammatory skin condition with a significant impact on patients' quality of life. Fumaric acid esters (FAEs) are amongst the first-line treatments in European countries where this medication is available. FAE are effective and generally safe but take a while to start working. Whereas the monotherapy with FAEs may take longer time to act, the combination with other therapies may accelerate the therapeutic response.

This randomized prospective clinical study was performed to assess the synergistic effect of a 6-week course of narrowband ultraviolet B therapy (NB-UVB) phototherapy in addition to FAE in adults with moderate-to-severe plaque psoriasis.

In this study, psoriasis patients with >10% BSA affected were chosen and randomized to either monotherapy with FAE or combination of FAE with NB-UVB. The primary outcome parameter was reduction in Psoriasis Area Severity Index (PASI) after 6 weeks of therapy. In addition, PASI 75 response (≥75% improvement from baseline PASI), the Psoriasis Log-based Area and Severity Index (PLASI) and the Dermatology Life Quality Index (DLQI) were assessed as secondary outcome measures.

In total, 30 patients were analyzed. The mean reduction in PASI after 6 weeks was significantly greater with the combination treatment than with FAE monotherapy. This was accompanied by a much faster improvement in the DLQI in the combination group than in the FAE-monotherapy group.

Key Message

- ***Combination therapy rather than monotherapy with FAE helps in comparatively faster disease clearance and improves the quality of life in psoriasis patients.***

ARTICLE 27

Association between Obesity and Pediatric Psoriasis

Hunjan MK, Maradit Kremers H, Lohse C, et al. Association between obesity and pediatric psoriasis. ***Pediatr Dermatol. 2018;35(5):e304-e305.***

Abstract

Obesity has been correlated with high risk of inception of psoriasis as well as with increased severity of psoriasis. At the time of diagnosis, obesity and psoriasis is seen. Here it is postulated that obesity precedes psoriasis.

COMMENT

This article studied the relationship between pediatric psoriasis and obesity. Psoriasis is commonly associated with metabolic syndrome in adults. Increased production of adipocytokines in central obesity leads to systemic inflammation and might thus lead to psoriasis.

This study shows that even in children, obesity increases the risk of developing psoriasis in children and moreover the severity of obesity correlates with the severity of psoriasis. This study also proposes that obesity might have preceded psoriasis even though obesity and psoriasis were coexisted at the time of diagnosis.

Children having psoriasis have higher risk of obesity, hyperlipidemia, diabetes, hypertension, polycystic ovarian disease, metabolic syndrome, elevated liver function tests and non-alcoholic liver disease in comparison to children without psoriasis. Having a parent who is overweight also increases the risk for psoriasis. Increased body mass index (BMI) is also associated with increased severity of psoriasis.

Thus, weight reduction may help in reducing the severity of psoriasis in obese children. This will also help to prevent other comorbidities related to obesity in the future which may further aggravate psoriasis independently such as diabetes, hypertension and hyperlipidemia.

A large-scale study with lipid levels, body mass index, body fat levels compared with the Psoriasis Area Severity Index (PASI) would be helpful. It would also be useful to study if there is reduction in severity or resolution of psoriasis after weight reduction.

Key Messages

- ***Children with obesity have higher risk of developing psoriasis and also have increased severity of the disease***
- ***Obesity may even precede development of psoriasis in children.***

ARTICLE 28

Real-world Health Outcomes in Adults with Moderate-to-Severe Psoriasis in the United States: A Population Study Using Electronic Health Records to Examine Patient-perceived Treatment Effectiveness, Medication Use, and Healthcare Resource Utilization

Armstrong AW, Foster SA, Comer BS, et al. Real-world health outcomes in adults with moderate-to-severe psoriasis in the United States: A population study using electronic health records to examine patient-perceived treatment effectiveness, medication use, and healthcare resource utilization.
BMC Dermatol. 2018;18(1):4.

Abstract

Electronic health records help to collect structured data and help to study the real-world outcomes in psoriasis patients. It helps to study the patient perception of medication usage, resource utilization, cost of medication and patient perception of effectiveness of treatment. In this study, more than 500,000 psoriasis patients were studied using electronic health records.

COMMENT

This article is a retrospective, longitudinal, multicenter, observational cohort study on patients of mild-to-moderate psoriasis in the United States using electronic health records (EHRs). It assessed the patterns of medication usage such as duration, switching or discontinuation of medication, medication cost. De-identification of data was done for ensuring patient privacy.

Body surface area involvement and static physician's global assessment (sPGA) were used to identify the disease severity. A score of ≥3 was considered to be moderate to severe disease. A pre-defined questionnaire was used to assess the patient perception on treatment effectiveness. The treatment groups into which patients were categorized for analyses were topical treatment, oral systemic treatments (acitretin, methotrexate, apremilast and cyclosporin), phototherapy, biologic treatment (secukinumab, etanercept, infliximab, adalimumab, or ustekinumab), combination treatments and other interventions (patients who were not on any of the above treatments).

The patients who were most satisfied with the treatment were those who were on biologics and those with good treatment adherence. The most common cause for discontinuation of oral systemic agents were side effects and of biologics was decreased efficacy which may result from formation of antibodies against the agent. Healthcare utilization was highest for phototherapy due to the frequent visits which are needed for this treatment. Annual medication cost was higher in biologics in comparison to oral systemic agents. Patients treated with combination therapy had treatment switching more than monotherapy patients.

Dermatology specific EHR helps in reducing the risk of misclassification since dermatology providers enter data. Data provided by dermatologists have a higher positive predictive rate.

Thus, maintaining specialty specific EHRs is useful in finding treatment patterns, adherence to treatment and the cost factors involved and this would help to give optimum treatment to patients assessing various factors.

Key Messages

- *Research using electronic health records helped in finding treatment patterns, effectiveness of treatment, reasons for switching treatment or discontinuing treatment, health resource utilization, treatment duration, patient satisfaction and treatment cost*
- *Widely implemented electronic health records by specialists can be implemented to aid in patient and clinician decisions in the management of psoriasis.*

ARTICLE 29

Dietary Recommendations for Adults with Psoriasis or Psoriatic Arthritis from the Medical Board of the National Psoriasis Foundation: A Systematic Review

Ford AR, Siegel M, Bagel J, et al. Dietary recommendations for adults with psoriasis or psoriatic arthritis from the medical board of the national psoriasis foundation: A systematic review.
***JAMA Dermatol.* 2018;154(8):934-50.**

Abstract

Psoriasis is an inflammatory disorder which has a chronic course and has a significant effect on the quality of life. Dietary advice is generally given in case of chronic disorders especially when associated with metabolic syndrome. A literature review of 55 studies with a total of 4534 patients with psoriasis were analyzed and based on these dietary recommendations for psoriasis were given.

COMMENT

This article is a systematic review on the dietary recommendations for psoriasis and psoriatic arthritis from the National Psoriasis foundation's medical board. Previous systematic reviews and literature from the MEDLINE database talking about the role of diet in psoriasis was taken for this review. Based on this evidence, dietary recommendations were made which were further voted on by the Medical Board of the National Psoriasis Foundation.

The role between psoriasis and metabolic syndrome is well known and there have been many studies stating the role of obesity in the inception and aggravation of psoriasis.

This review was based on 55 studies having 4534 patients of psoriasis and a total of 77557 participants. Dietary weight reduction with a hypocaloric diet is recommended in obese and overweight psoriatic patients. If gluten sensitivity is present, a gluten free diet was advised. In addition, vitamin D supplementation along with weight reduction and a hypocaloric diet was recommended in psoriatic arthritis.

However, dietary interventions need to be combined with standard medical treatment for psoriasis and psoriatic arthritis and it will only act as a supplementary measure and not as a stand-alone therapy.

Moreover, all the dietary interventions will also reduce the other comorbidities of psoriasis such as diabetes mellitus, hypertension and hyperlipidemia and these in turn will help to reduce the severity of the disease.

Key Messages

- ***Dietary weight reduction and a hypocaloric diet helps to reduce the severity of psoriasis and psoriatic arthritis. In addition, vitamin D supplementation has proven to be of benefit in psoriatic arthritis***
- ***Dietary interventions have to be combined with standard medical therapies for the management of psoriasis and psoriatic arthritis.***

ARTICLE 30

Turmeric Tonic as a Treatment in Scalp Psoriasis: A Randomized Placebo-control Clinical Trial

Bahraini P, Rajabi M, Mansouri P, et al. Turmeric tonic as a treatment in scalp psoriasis: A randomized placebo-control clinical trial.
J Cosmet Dermatol. 2018;17(3):461-6.

Abstract

Psoriasis is a chronic inflammatory disorder having a strong genetic predisposition. Scalp is one of the most common areas affected. This is usually treated with topical steroids which are associated with various side effects. Turmeric which is used as a spice has anti-inflammatory, antineoplastic, antioxidant and antimicrobial properties. It also has an inhibitory activity on potassium channels in T cells. In this study, turmeric tonic showed significant benefit in the treatment of scalp psoriasis.

COMMENT

This article is a study on the immunomodulatory and anti-inflammatory use of turmeric tonic in scalp psoriasis. Scalp psoriasis is usually treated with topical steroids, coal tar and salicylic acid-based shampoos. The former on long-term usage could lead to various adverse effects.

Turmeric the biologic name of which is *Curcuma longa L.* is a spice which is used widely in India. Women generally apply it over the body while taking bath. It is also applied over wounds commonly. It is presumed to have antimicrobial, anti-inflammatory, antineoplastic and antioxidant properties.

Turmeric (*Curcuma longa L.*), a spice commonly used throughout the world has been reported to exhibit inhibitory activity on potassium channels in T cells and plays a key role in psoriasis.

This was a randomized control trial with a sample size of 40. The case group were given turmeric tonic to be applied twice a day for a period of nine weeks and the control group received a placebo. Evaluation was done at baseline, 3, 6 and 9 weeks. Pre and post treatment photographs, Psoriasis Area Severity Index (PASI) and Dermatology Life Quality Index (DLQI) scores were assessed.

Significant improvement was found in the PASI and DLQI scores in the turmeric tonic group compared to the placebo group with a p-value of <0.05 which is significant indicating that turmeric tonic could be used as a treatment for scalp psoriasis.

Turmeric is traditionally used as a method of hair reduction in south Indian women which is why it is frequently applied over the body. It may be difficult to convince the patients to apply it over the scalp. Yellowish staining of the hair and scalp may also not be cosmetically acceptable to the patient.

Turmeric has been long self-used by patients for a variety of skin conditions including acne and dermatophytosis. Turmeric used as a treatment modality by a qualified specialist may further incite the patients to believe and use this solution for a variety of skin disorders.

A larger study with a greater sample size, double blinding and a longer follow-up is required to consider prescribing turmeric tonic for scalp psoriasis. Moreover, apart from DLQI, the patient satisfaction on the treatment efficacy could also be assessed.

Key Messages

- *Turmeric reduces the severity of lesions in psoriasis as compared to psoriasis*
- *Turmeric tonic could be used as a treatment for scalp psoriasis to avoid the side effects of long-term steroid usage.*

ARTICLE 31

Prevalence of Psoriatic Arthritis in Patients with Psoriasis: A Systematic Review and Meta-analysis of Observational and Clinical Studies

Alinaghi F, Calov M, Kristensen LE, et al. Prevalence of psoriatic arthritis in patients with psoriasis: A systematic review and meta-analysis of observational and clinical studies.
J Am Acad Dermatol. 2018;S0190-9622(18):32149-2.

Abstract

Psoriatic arthritis is widely prevalent in patients with psoriasis. This study analyzed the prevalence of psoriatic arthritis in patients with psoriasis. Three databases were searched by two authors and a meta-analysis was conducted. A total of 266 studies having 976,408 patients were studied.

COMMENT

This article is a review and analysis of observational and clinical studies reporting the incidence and prevalence of psoriatic arthritis (PsA) in patients with psoriasis. Two authors went through three databases for this purpose and a pooled meta-analysis was done. This was a retrospective observational study.

A total of 97,6408 patients were studied from a total of 266 studies. About 19.7% of patients with psoriasis had PsA. In a study where CASPAR (ClASsification criteria for Psoriatic ARthritis) criteria was used to diagnose PsA, the prevalence of PsA was 23.8%. The highest prevalence of PsA in psoriasis was in Europeans (22.7%) and the lowest was in Asians (14%). Psoriatic patients less than 18 years of age had a 3.3% prevalence of PsA.

The incidence of PsA in psoriatic patients varied in different studies and ranged from 0.27 to 2.7 per 100 person-years.

Since the incidence of PsA in psoriasis patients is less in childhood and adolescence, duration of the disease may also play a role in the development of PsA. Hence, a data on the duration of the disease with the prevalence of PsA in psoriasis patients also can be done.

Comparison of the severity of psoriasis with the help of psoriatic arthritis screening and evaluation (PASE) and Psoriasis Area Severity Index (PASI), and Nail Psoriasis Severity Index (NAPSI) can also be done.

Classification criteria for psoriatic arthritis score was used in only certain studies and not all of them. The basis on which the diagnosis of PsA was done in other patients has not been mentioned.

Further studies where CASPAR score is used to identify all patients with PsA in patients with psoriasis would be helpful.

This study also highlights the use of proper data maintenance in doing various observational studies on psoriasis patients.

Key Messages

- ***Psoriatic arthritis was present in 19.7% of patients with psoriasis***
- ***With the advent of CASPAR and PASE scores in studies, reporting of a higher prevalence rate can be expected.***

ARTICLE 32

A Multicenter, Prospective, Observational Study Examining the Impact of Risk Factors, Such as BMI and Waist Circumference, on Quality of Life Improvement and Clinical Response in Moderate-to-Severe Plaque-type Psoriasis Patients Treated with Infliximab in Routine Care Settings of Greece

Petridis A, Panagaksis P, Moustou E, et al. A multicenter, prospective, observational study examining the impact of risk factors, such as BMI and waist circumference, on quality of life improvement and clinical response in moderate-to-severe plaque-type psoriasis patients treated with infliximab in routine care settings of Greece.
J Eur Acad Dermatol Venereol. 2018;32(5):768-75.

Abstract

Obesity has a correlation with the severity of moderate-to-severe plaque psoriasis and with treatment response of biologic therapies. In this study, 136 patients with a BMI of 29.6 and waist circumference of 107 cm were taken. All the patients had received treatment for psoriasis but were biologic naïve. Patients were treated with infliximab and followed up at 14, 30 and 54 weeks. The effect of BMI and waist circumference on the treatment response and the quality of life was studied.

COMMENT

This article is a study on the effect of body mass index (BMI) and waist circumference (WC) on the quality of life and clinical improvement of moderate-to-severe plaque psoriasis treated with infliximab.

In other studies, obesity has known to have a relation in precipitating and aggravating psoriasis and has shown to have a relation with moderate-to-severe psoriasis. It also shown to have an effect on PASI 75 (75 reduction in psoriasis area severity index) attainment of biologic therapies.

This study was an observational multicenter prospective study conducted in Greece. The parameters studied were the effect of BMI and WC on the disease severity, the patient characteristics associated with clinical response and improvement in health-related quality of life (HRQoL) on treatment with infliximab.

Patients of moderate-to-severe psoriasis who were treated with infliximab for 2 weeks were enrolled for the study. Subsequent data were collected at 14 ± 4, 30 ± 4 and 54 ± 4 weeks after treatment.

A total of 136 patients were studied by 21 dermatologists. A low correlation was observed between the WC and PASI score at enrolment. A total of 89.3% patients achieved a PASI 75 at a median of 48.4 weeks of treatment. Greater than or equal to 5-point Dermatology Life Quality Index (DLQI) decrease (considered to be clinically meaningful) and PASI 75 at 54 weeks of treatment were 69.8% and 76.6% respectively.

Waist circumference and BMI at enrolment did not affect the PASI 75 or DLQI improvement.

Most of the studies have shown a decreased response to treatment in psoriasis patients with obesity. Even though this study shows an increased WC relation to the PASI score on enrolment, it did not show decrease of treatment response in obese patients. Further studies are needed to confirm this finding.

In other studies weight reduction has been shown to improve the treatment response and severity of psoriasis. This study suggests taking BMI and WC only at the beginning of the study. Only the other parameters such as PASI 75 and decrease in DLQI were measured at the follow-ups. It is suggested to take it at the end of the study, since a decrease in those parameters might have also contributed to treatment response.

Key Messages

- ***Infliximab improved the disease activity and quality of life of patients with moderate-to-severe psoriasis in 1 year of treatment***
- ***There was effect on BMI and WC on the response to treatment.***

ARTICLE 33

A Multidimensional Assessment of the Burden of Psoriasis: Results from a Multinational Dermatologist and Patient Survey

Griffiths CEM, Jo SJ, Naldi L, et al. A multidimensional assessment of the burden of psoriasis: Results from a multinational dermatologist and patient survey.
Br J Dermatol. 2018;179(1):173-81.

Abstract

Psoriasis is a chronic immune mediated inflammatory disorder which has a significant negative impact on the quality of life, cost burden and work productivity. A multinational survey was done using data from the Growth from knowledge disease atlas global real-world evidence program. The effect of other psychological comorbidities, physical and psychological comorbidities, itch and sensitive and visible body area involvement on the work impairment and quality of life was assessed.

COMMENT

This article is a study on the effect of factors like itching, visible body area involvement, physical and psychological comorbidities on the work productivity and quality of life (QoL) in patients of moderate and severe psoriasis.

It was a multinational observational study and studied 3,821 patients of psoriasis in nine countries with the help of 524 dermatologists.

Dermatologists with over 3-year experience post-training and those who see at least 10 psoriasis patients of psoriasis per week and those who were responsible for making treatment decisions were recruited for conducting the study. Adult patients with psoriasis above 18 years who has moderate-to-severe psoriasis (physician assessed) were taken for the study. The patients completed a survey after the consultation.

Dermatologists reported psoriasis symptoms (presence and extent of itch, sleep disturbance due to itch, skin pain), medical resource utilization in the last 1 year (number of visits with the dermatologist, history of admissions, involvement of any other physician such as a rheumatologist in the patient's management) and the extent of the skin disease (PASI score) and the areas involved. The patients filled forms of Dermatology Life Quality Index (DLQI), short form health survey (SF-12), EuroQol-5 Dimensions questionnaire (EQ-5D) and work productivity and activity impairment (WPAI).

The patients were separated into groups on the basis of presence and severity of the itch, those with and without comorbidities such as obesity, type 2 diabetes, psoriatic arthritis, anxiety or depression and cardiovascular involvement and also on the areas involved (visible vs. covered areas). All models were matched for effects of demographics (gender, age body mass index, country of origin, alcohol intake and smoking), time since diagnosis and the treatment received, psoriasis severity, current PASI score and the number of exacerbations in the last 1 year.

Associated comorbidities increased the chance of skin pain, lower QoL, work impairment and increase in use of resources (especially other specialty consultation in psoriatic arthritis). Those with visible body area involvement and itch also had a lower QoL in comparison to those without these features.

Key Messages

- ***The clinical, economic, and humanistic burden of psoriasis is just not dependent on the severity of the disease***
- ***There is a significant role of having visible skin lesions, itching and other psychological and physical comorbidities in the quality of life and work impairment in psoriasis patients.***

ARTICLE 34

A Systematic Review and Meta-analysis of Efficacy and Safety of Novel Interleukin Inhibitors in the Management of Psoriatic Arthritis

Bilal J, Riaz IB, Kamal MU, et al. A systematic review and meta-analysis of efficacy and safety of novel interleukin inhibitors in the management of psoriatic arthritis.
J Clin Rheumatol. 2018;24(1):6-13.

Abstract

Interleukin inhibitors such as clazakizumab, ustekinumab, brodalumab, ixekizumab and secukinumab are used in the treatment of psoriasis and psoriatic arthritis. This study analysed the safety and efficacy of these agents in the treatment of psoriatic arthritis. Literature search was done using web of science, Scopus, Cochrane library, MEDLINE and EMBASE. American College of Rheumatology 20 response was studied at 24 weeks.

COMMENT

This article is a review and analysis on the effectiveness and safety of interleukin inhibitors in the treatment of psoriatic arthritis (PsA). The interleukin inhibitors studied were clazakizumab (IL-6 inhibitor), secukinumab, brodalumab, and ixekizumab (IL-17A inhibitor) and ustekinumab (IL-12/23 inhibitor).

Studies which showed an American College of Rheumatology (ACR) 20 response at 24 weeks were also included. ACR 20 is defined as 20% improvement in the number of tender and swollen joints and also 20% improvement in three of the following five criteria including physician global assessment, patient global assessment, visual analog pain scale, erythrocyte sedimentation rate or C-reactive protein and health assessment questionnaire.

A total of 2,722 patients in eight studies were reviewed. There was a significant improvement in ACR ratios in all the drugs studies compared to placebo. There was not much difference in the results of different studies. Subgroup analysis in patients who were tumor necrosis factor (TNF) naïve and TNF non-responders or inadequate responders also showed results with the IL inhibitors. The side effects were more in the drug group compared to placebo though not severe enough to stop medication. There was not much of significant worsening on drug withdrawal.

Though this is a review, mainly conducted for the efficacy of IL inhibitors in PsA, a similar review can be done for the improvement of skin lesions with IL inhibitors.

Improvement in the Psoriasis Area Severity Index (PASI) and Nail Psoriasis Severity Index (NAPSI) score can be assessed and the period of remission on drug withdrawal can be assessed. Psoriatic arthritis screening and evaluation (PASE) scores can also be done apart from the ACR response to see if there is an improvement with treatment.

Key Message

- ***Interleukin inhibitors such as secukinumab, brodalumab, ixekizumab, clazakizumab and ustekinumab are well tolerated and effective in the treatment of psoriatic arthritis.***

ARTICLE 35

Analysis of Anti-tumour Necrosis Factor-induced Skin Lesions Reveals Strong T Helper 1 Activation with some Distinct Immunological Characteristics

Stoffel E, Maier H, Riedl E, et al. Analysis of anti-tumour necrosis factor-induced skin lesions reveals strong T helper 1 activation with some distinct immunological characteristics.
Br J Dermatol. 2018;178(5):1151-62.

Abstract

Tumor necrosis factor-α inhibitor therapy causes dermatological reactions such as psoriasiform and eczematous reactions. This study analyzed the histopathological, cellular and molecular features of these reactions and compared it with those of eczema, psoriasis and healthy control skin. It was found out that this entity was different on all the levels from eczema to psoriasis and is a separate entity.

COMMENT

This article is a study on the skin lesions induced by anti-tumor necrosis factor (TNF)-α therapy and comparing them on a cellular, histopathological and molecular basis to psoriasis, eczema and normal control skin.

The common skin lesions associated with anti-TNF therapy include psoriasiform eczema, eczema, psoriasis, xerosis and palmoplantar pustulosis.

In this study, skin biopsies from new onset inflammatory skin lesions from 19 patients on anti-TNF-α therapy for rheumatoid arthritis and inflammatory bowel disease were taken. Histopathological evaluation, computer assisted immunohistochemical studies (Tissue FAXS- an upright fluorescence and brightfield system for the scanning and analysis of slides, cytospins, smears and tissue microarrays) and gene expression (quantitative real-time polymerase chain reaction) were done on the biopsies. These same characteristics were compared to biopsies of psoriasis, eczema and normal skin.

The histopathological features of the patients on anti-TNF-α therapy showed either spongiotic (suggestive of eczema) changes or psoriasiform changes or both. However on a molecular level the lesions were not suggestive of neither psoriasis nor eczema. Moreover, all the anti-TNF-α-induced lesions showed a higher interferon (IFN)-γ activation compared to both eczema and psoriasis.

This suggests that even though clinically and histopathologically anti-TNF-α-induced lesions may resemble eczema or psoriasis or both, on a molecular and a cellular level these lesions are different.

A study on a larger group of patients would be useful to confirm this finding although it would be quite expensive to perform molecular and cellular studies on a large cohort of patients.

It remains to be known whether certain other reactions to drugs which resemble skin disorders like psoriasis, lichen planus and dermatitis are different from these conditions on a molecular and cellular basis.

Key Messages

- ***The skin lesions of patients on anti-TNF-α therapy though they resemble psoriasis, eczema or both clinically and histopathologically, they show different molecular and cellular characteristics***
- ***Hence, skin lesions have to be considered as a different entity to psoriasis and/or eczema.***

ARTICLE 36

Association between Circulating Prolactin Levels and Psoriasis and Its Correlation with Disease Severity: A Meta-analysis

Lee YH, Song GG. Association between circulating prolactin levels and psoriasis and its correlation with disease severity: A meta-analysis.
Clin Exp Dermatol. 2018;43(1):27-35.

Abstract

Various studies have been done to compare circulating prolactin levels with the severity of psoriasis with variable results. A total of 12 studies having 446 psoriasis patients and 401 controls were analyzed. The prolactin levels were compared in the psoriasis and the healthy control group and the severity of the disease on the basis of PASI score was compared with the prolactin levels. Psoriasis patients had a higher prolactin level compared to controls and the severity of the disease also correlated with the prolactin levels.

COMMENT

This article is a meta-analysis of the circulating serum prolactin levels with psoriasis disease severity. A total of 12 studies having a total of 446 psoriasis patients and 401 healthy controls (HCs) were included in the analysis.

The serum and plasma levels of prolactin in both the psoriasis and HCs were compared. The correlation between serum prolactin levels and the psoriasis severity assessed by means of Psoriasis Area Severity Index (PASI) score was also assessed.

Prolactin levels were significantly higher in the psoriasis group as compared to the HC group in stratification by age and sex. There was a correlation between PASI score and prolactin levels though it was not statistically significant ($p = 0.08 > 0.05$)

Estrogen is known to promote a conversion of the immune response from Th1 to Th2 type. Prolactin is also known to have a similar effect. Hence, these hormones should technically have a protective role in psoriasis and an adverse effect in atopic dermatitis and connective tissue disorders.

Prolactin exhibits a proliferative effect on cultured human keratinocytes and increases *in vitro* production of vascular endothelial growth factor (VEGF). Thus, it may stimulate keratinocyte proliferation and promote angiogenesis. It also inhibits suppressor T cells. interferon (IFN)-γ production by prolactin may induce secretion of chemokines such as CXCL9, CXCL10 and CXCL11.

Bromocriptine which is potent dopaminergic inhibitor of pituitary prolactin secretion has been known to have remission of skin lesions of psoriasis and psoriatic arthritis.

Further studies and analysis on levels of prolactin in psoriasis is necessary to use prolactin inhibitors as a mode of treatment in psoriasis.

Key Messages

- ***Prolactin levels are significantly higher in psoriasis patients as compared to healthy controls***
- ***There is a non-statistically significant correlation between the PASI score and the prolactin levels.***

ARTICLE 37

Burden of Chronic Urticaria Relative to Psoriasis in Five European Countries

Balp MM, Khalil S, Tian H, et al. Burden of chronic urticaria relative to psoriasis in five European countries.
J Eur Acad Dermatol Venereol. 2018;32(2):282-90.

Abstract

The quantification of burden of chronic spontaneous urticaria (CSU) with that of psoriasis is limited. The objective of this study was to assess the burden of CSU with psoriasis overall as well as with mild and moderate-to-severe psoriasis. This study was conducted with data from five countries. The parameters studied were mental and physical component scores, activity impairment, work productivity and self-reported healthcare utilization. A total of 769 CSU patients and 7,857 psoriasis patients were studied. The burden of CSU was more when compared to psoriasis overall but was similar to that of moderate-to-severe psoriasis though both conditions had the same negative impact on work productivity.

COMMENT

This article is an analysis of data and comparison of the burden of chronic spontaneous urticaria (CSU) overall with that of psoriasis in general as well as separately with moderate/severe psoriasis.

Data were taken from National health and wellness survey in five countries namely Germany, France, Spain, United Kingdom and Italy. The parameters studied were mental and physical component summary scores, self-reported psychological complaints and health resource utilization and work impairment. Analysis for each outcome was done with comparative groups.

A total of 7,857 psoriasis patients of which 26.9% was moderate/severe psoriasis and 769 CSU patients were studied.

Chronic spontaneous urticaria patients showed a greater impairment in the Quality of Life (QoL), healthcare utilization and a higher risk of psychological comorbidities compared to psoriasis patients overall. Impact on work outcome was similar in both the groups. However, all these parameters were similar to patients of moderate/severe psoriasis.

Both psoriasis and CSU are chronic disorders which significantly impair the QoL of patients, causes psychological disturbances and need treatment for long duration of time using significant amount of health resources.

In this study, a significantly larger number of psoriasis patients were studied compared to psoriasis patients. Both the sample sizes should be similar if not same to consider the result valid. The different degrees of urticaria could also be noted down since the extent of psoriasis was noted down. It is suggested to compare mild urticaria and mild psoriasis and severe urticaria with moderate/severe psoriasis. The duration of both the diseases could also be noted and the parameters compared with the duration of each disorder.

Key Message

- ***The burden of chronic urticaria is more as compared to psoriasis of all grades, but similar to what is seen in moderate and severe psoriasis.***

ARTICLE 38

Biologics Combined with Conventional Systemic Agents or Phototherapy for the Treatment of Psoriasis: Real-life Data from PSONET Registries

Busard CI, Cohen AD, Wolf P, et al. Biologics combined with conventional systemic agents or phototherapy for the treatment of psoriasis: real-life data from PSONET registries.

J Eur Acad Dermatol Venereol. 2018;32(2):245-53.

Abstract

Biologics are commonly used for the management of psoriasis. However, primary and secondary non-response to treatment is seen which needs better strategies to improve outcome. The objective of this study was to describe combination treatment of biologics with systemic agents or phototherapy.

Data on the frequency of use, treatment characteristics, drug survival and treatment characteristics in combination with conventional systemic therapies or phototherapy was analyzed from five PSONET registries. A total of 9,922 biologic treatments were studied. About 982 were combination treatment out of which methotrexate was the most common combination followed by ultraviolet B (UVB) therapy, acitretin and cyclosporin. Methotrexate also had the highest survival in combination with biologics again followed by acitretin and cyclosporin.

COMMENT

This article is a collection of data to describe the combination of biologics with other lines of therapy such as phototherapy and conventional systemic therapy in daily practice.

Biologics have greatly improved psoriasis management. However, primary and secondary non-response to treatment requires innovative strategies to optimize outcomes.

Data of demographics, frequency of use, treatment characteristics, drug survival (length of time until discontinuation of the drug) of biologics combined with phototherapy and other systemic agents were studied. Data were taken from five PSONET registries which is a network of independent European, population-based registries of patients having psoriasis and psoriatic arthritis.

A total of 9922 biologic treatment cycles were studied. Out of that 9.9% (982) were identified as combination treatment. Out of these 982, 72.9% cycles had concomitant use of methotrexate, concomitant ultraviolet B (UVB) therapy, cyclosporin or acitretin was seen in 25.3% cases and 1.8% had concomitant therapy with a second biologic, psoralen and ultraviolet A (PUVA) or fumaric acids.

There was a significant variation in the frequency and type of combination treatments across various registries. The patients who were initiated on combination therapy generally had severe disease and a longer duration of the disease.

There was no consistent superior survival for one particular biologic. Longest survival rate of biologics was seen when combined with methotrexate.

It is advised to combine biologics with another line of treatment especially in severe psoriasis. Moreover, primary and secondary non-response to treatment may occur with biologics which need to be combated by using combination treatments.

The increased cost of biologics also makes combination treatments more viable. This could also probably be the reason of the survival rates combinations with methotrexate being high, as it is cost-effective compared to cyclosporine and acitretin.

Methotrexate was the most commonly used concomitant treatment for patients on a biologic. Wide geographical variations in treatment selection and persistence of combination treatment exist. Data derived from ongoing studies may help to determine whether combined treatment is superior to biologic monotherapy.

Key Messages

- ***The most commonly used concomitant treatment for patients on biologic therapy for psoriasis was methotrexate***
- ***There is a wide geographical variation in selection of treatment and combination treatment for psoriasis***
- ***Biologics have brought a great improvement to the management of psoriasis. However, non-response to treatment, needs combination treatment to improve outcome.***

ARTICLE 39

Carboxytherapy for Treatment of Localized Chronic Plaque Psoriasis: Clinical and Histopathologic Evaluation

Kamel AM, Abdelghani R. Carboxytherapy for treatment of localized chronic plaque psoriasis: Clinical and histopathologic evaluation.
J Cosmet Dermatol. 2018;17(3):527-32.

Abstract

Multiple modalities have been used for the treatment of localized chronic plaque psoriasis but with poor patient satisfaction and outcome. The objective of this pilot study was to assess the safety and efficacy of carboxytherapy in the treatment of localized chronic plaque psoriasis. 30 patients were administered injections of carboxytherapy weekly for 8 weeks. Histopathological and clinical evaluation was done, a fortnight after the last injection. The parameters studied were total sign score, 5-point scale for perilesional erythema and investigators global assessment. The recurrence was studied 3 months following the ultimate session using a 10-point scale. Treatment success was seen in 26.6% of patients and perilesional erythema disappeared in 70% of the patients.

COMMENT

This article is a study on the use of carboxytherapy for the management of localized chronic plaque psoriasis.

Carboxytherapy is the controlled application or injection of purified carbon dioxide into various areas. It improves the blood circulation, improves elasticity and reduces fat deposition in tissues.

Thirty patients having localized chronic plaque psoriasis were taken for the study. They were treated with carboxytherapy injections once per week for a period of 8 weeks. The parameters evaluated were 10-point visual analog scale assessing patient satisfaction, total sign score, investigators global assessment and 5- point scale for perilesional erythema. Clinical and histopathological evaluation was done 2 weeks after the last treatment and evaluation for recurrence was done with the help of a 10-point scale 3 months after the last session.

According to investigator's global assessment and total sign score, carboxytherapy had achieved success in 26.6% of cases. Absence of perilesional erythema was seen in 70% of cases. No side effects were sent with full patient satisfaction. 83.3% of the patients who had improvement showed recurrence within 1–10% of the baseline area.

Therefore, increased frequency of sessions may be needed to reduce recurrence. It cannot be used for extensive psoriasis but can be used for some resistant plaques in extensive disease. The cost of the treatment may prove to be a limiting factor.

Key Message

- ***Carboxytherapy will be useful in localised lesions of psoriasis if the number of sessions of the therapy are increased and the regular sessions are followed by maintainable sessions.***

ARTICLE 40

Comparison of Effectiveness and Safety of Excimer Lamp Vs Topical Calcipotriol-clobetasol Propionate Combination in the Treatment of Palmoplantar Psoriasis

Thakur A, Bishnoi A, Dogra S, et al. Comparison of effectiveness and safety of excimer lamp vs topical calcipotriol-clobetasol propionate combination in the treatment of palmoplantar psoriasis.
Photodermatol Photoimmunol Photomed. 2018;34(4):249-56.

Abstract

The efficacy of excimer laser in the treatment of palmoplantar psoriasis (PPP) has not been determined. The purpose of this study was to compare the efficacy and safety of excimer laser with topical calcipotriol-clobetasol combination in PPP. A left-right randomization was done with 36 patients where one side was treated twice weekly with excimer lamp and the other with clobetasol-calcipotriol combination once daily applied. The parameters studied were improvement in palmoplantar pustular psoriasis area and severity index score. Both excimer laser and the calcipotriol-clobetasol combination were proven to be equally effective in the treatment of PPP.

COMMENT

This article is a study which aimed to ascertain the safety and efficacy of excimer laser in comparison to a topical ointment made of calcipotriol (0.005%) and clobetasol propionate (0.05%) in patients with palmoplantar psoriasis (PPP).

This was a right-left randomized trial done with 36 patients having PPP. The patients received excimer laser treatment twice weekly on one side and the clobetasol-calcipotriol combination once in a day on the other side. The treatment was given for a period of 12 weeks and follow-up was continued for a period of 8 weeks after the treatment.

The response was assessed by two dermatologists. The parameters assessed were mPPASI (modified palmoplantar pustular psoriasis area and severity index score). The outcome assessed at the end of 2 weeks were classified as minimal (≤25%), mild (>25–50%), moderate (>50–75%), and marked (>75%). The proportion of patients achieving >75% reduction in mPPASI and the time required for it was also assessed.

Excimer lasers deliver a high intensity ultraviolet B (UVB) light of a specific wavelength (308 nm) aimed directly at the psoriatic plaques. It works faster (fewer sessions are required and a stronger light which can penetrate deeper can be used) than traditional light therapy. The hand-held laser is also useful for accessing hard to reach areas such as palms, soles, scalp, elbows and knees. The side effects commonly associated include pigmentation (hypo or hyper), purpura, erythema, pruritus, burning, blistering and scarring. However, using topical steroid based ointments for a long duration can also cause hypopigmentation and telangiectasias.

Among the 36 recruited patients, 33 finished treatment (12 weeks) and 21 came for the 8 weeks follow-up. The mPPASI reduced significantly post treatment with both the treatments and the reduction was not significantly different among the two groups. The side effects (most commonly hyperpigmentation) were more in the excimer treated group but it was not significant enough to halt treatment. The mPPASI 75 in 2, 4, and 8 weeks in 1, 2, and 8 patients respectively.

Since the effects of both treatments are equal, they can be used alternatively to minimize the side effects of each of them.

A longer duration study is required to assess the long-term benefit and adverse effects of both the treatments.

Key Messages

- *Excimer lamp and calcipotriol-clobetasol propionate combination both are equally effective for treatment of palmoplantar psoriasis*
- *The adverse effects (most common of which was hyperpigmentation) were seen more in the excimer treated sites.*

ARTICLE 41

Comparison of Indirubin Concentrations in *Indigo naturalis* Ointment for Psoriasis Treatment: A Randomized, Double-blind, Dosage-controlled Trial

Lin YK, See LC, Huang YH, et al. Comparison of indirubin concentrations in *Indigo naturalis* ointment for psoriasis treatment: A randomized, double-blind, dosage-controlled trial.
Br J Dermatol. 2018;178(1):124-31.

Abstract

Indigo naturalis is a useful topical treatment for psoriasis. Lindioil is its refined formulation. The active ingredient in *Indigo naturalis* is indirubin. The objective of this study was to study the efficacy and safety of different concentrations of indirubin in Lindioil ointment in the treatment of psoriasis. The concentrations studied were 10, 50, 100, 200 $\mu g\ g^{-1}$ of indirubin. It was applied twice daily for 8 weeks followed by a 12-week extension period. The endpoint studied was percentage change in PASI score and the proportion of patients achieving PASI 75 and PASI 90. The most effective and safe concentration was 200 µg/g of indirubin in Lindioil ointment.

COMMENT

The article is a study on the safety and efficacy of indirubin (the active ingredient in *Indigo naturalis*) in Lindioil ointment in treating psoriasis.

Indigo naturalis is a Chinese herb and is a dried pigment derived from various plant species including *Baphicacanthus cusia*. The anti-psoriatic effects of *Indigo naturalis* are mediated by modulating the proliferation and differentiation of keratinocytes, the major active component being indirubin. Indirubin inhibits cyclin-dependent kinase, signal transduction and activation of transcriptase-3 (STAT3) and also *in vitro* keratinocyte proliferation. Indirubin and indigo, both major components of *Indigo naturalis* cause G (0)/G (1) phase arrest, but only Indirubin modulated the effect of proliferating cell nuclear antigen (PCNA) and involucrin expression similar to the effect obtained by *Indigo naturalis*.

This was a randomized, double-blind study in which adult patients having chronic plaque psoriasis for a duration of more than a year and with less than 20% body surface area involvement were taken for the study. They were randomly split into groups and were given 10, 50, 100 or 200 µg/g of indirubin to be applied twice daily for a period of 2 months followed by a 3-month extension period.

The parameters measured were the mean change in Psoriasis Area Severity Index (PASI) score in each group and the proportion of patients in each group having 75% and 90% reduction in PASI score i.e. PASI 75 and PASI 90 respectively by week 8 of treatment.

The 200 µg/g group had the greatest reduction in PASI score and also has the highest proportion of patients achieving PASI 75 and PASI 90. No adverse effects were seen in the 5-month period of evaluation. The 100 µg/g group had the next best efficacy, but the efficacy of the 10 µg/g group was more than that of the 50 µg/g group.

The long-term side effects of the highest concentration use of indirubin needs to be studied. It needs to be studied if even higher concentrations improve the efficacy further or the effect plateau over a period of time. Moreover, it needs to be studied if there is any tachyphylaxis in this mode of treatment.

Key Message

- ***The most effective concentration of indirubin (an active ingredient of Indigo naturalis) in Lindioil ointment is 200 µg/g for psoriasis.***

ARTICLE 42

Efficacy and Safety of Tofacitinib for Moderate-to-Severe Plaque Psoriasis: A Systematic Review and Meta-analysis of Randomized Controlled Trials

Kuo CM, Tung TH, Wang SH, et al. Efficacy and safety of tofacitinib for moderate-to-severe plaque psoriasis: A systematic review and meta-analysis of randomized controlled trials.
J Eur Acad Dermatol Venereol. 2018;32(3):355-62.

Abstract

The aim of this study was to assess the effect of tofacitinib in the treatment of moderate-to-severe plaque psoriasis. Four randomized control trials with a total of 2,724 participants were selected through Cochrane Central Register of Controlled Trials, EMBASE and PubMed and a systematic review and meta-analysis was done. Tofacitinib showed significant improvement in the PASI score, Physician's Global Assessment and DLQI. Thus, in conclusion tofacitinib can be used as a treatment option in cases of moderate-to-severe plaque psoriasis in patients who do not tolerate other therapies or in those who prefer oral medication.

COMMENT

This article is a systematic review and meta-analysis of randomized controlled trials (RCTs) to study the effect of tofacitinib in treatment of moderate-to-severe psoriasis.

Tofacitinib is a targeted small molecule and an oral Janus Kinase inhibitor (JAK inhibitor) which helps to modulate cytokines which are necessary for progression of inflammatory and immune responses.

The cytoplasmic domain of type I and II cytokine receptors bind to members of kinase family referred to as Janus kinases (Jaks). The Jaks include Jak1, Jak2, Jak3 and Tyk2. Different cytokine receptors are paired with different Jaks which get activated on cytokine binding to cytokine receptors. The Jaks are phosphotransferases and catalyze transfer to phosphate from adenosine triphosphate (ATP) to substrates such as cytokine receptors.

Tofacitinib inhibits Jak1, Jak3 and to a lesser extent Jak2. Thus, all the cytokines signaled through Jak3 such as Interleukin (IL)-2, IL-4, IL-7, IL-9, IL-15, and IL-21 are blocked. Since it blocks Jak1, there is inhibition of gp130 family which includes IL-11 and IL-6 as well as IL-10, interferon (IFN)-α/β and IFN-γ. Since it blocks Jak2, it blocks IL-5, Il-3, granulocyte-macrophage colony-stimulating factor (GM-CSF) and IFN-γ.

Randomized control trials were collected from Cochrane Central Register of Controlled Trials, PubMed and EMBASE. A total of 2,724 participants were studied from four studies and systematic review, and meta-analysis was done.

There was a significant improvement in patients treated with tofacitinib compared to patients on placebo with achievement of PASI 75 (75% reduction in the PASI score). Both dosage of 5 mg BD and 10 mg BD gave significant results. There was an improvement in the Physician's global assessment and the Dermatology Life Quality Index.

There was an increase in minor adverse effects with both 5 mg and 10 mg dosage of tofacitinib. Upper respiratory tract infection and hypercholesterolemia were the most common adverse effects.

In conclusion, tofacitinib may be a treatment option for moderate-to-severe plaque psoriasis that is unresponsive to other therapies and patients who are intolerable to other therapies or prefer oral medications.

Key Message

- ***Tofacitinib, a Janus Kinase inhibitor is a treatment option for patients with moderate-to-severe plaque psoriasis who prefer oral medications and those who do not response or are not able to tolerate other therapies.***

ARTICLE 43

Efficacy and Safety of Guselkumab in Patients with Psoriasis Who Have an Inadequate Response to Ustekinumab: Results of the Randomized, Double-blind, Phase III NAVIGATE Trial

Langley RG, Tsai TF, Flavin S, et al. Efficacy and safety of guselkumab in patients with psoriasis who have an inadequate response to ustekinumab: Results of the randomized, double-blind, phase III NAVIGATE trial.
Br J Dermatol. 2018;178(1):114-23.

Abstract

Guselkumab is an anti-IL-23 monoclonal antibody which has exhibited good efficacy in phase III trials for psoriasis. The objective of this phase III trial was to assess the safety and efficacy of guselkumab in patients who had inadequate response to ustekinumab in moderate-to-severe plaque psoriasis. A total of 871 patients received ustekinumab and 268 who showed inadequate response at week 16 were randomized in a double-blind manner into two groups one of which received ustekinumab and the other guselkumab. The parameters assessed were number of weeks to achieve investigator global assessment of 0/1, PASI 90/100 and DLQI of 0/1. There was a significant benefit in shifting the patient to guselkumab in patients who did not respond to ustekinumab.

COMMENT

This article was a study to evaluate the efficacy of guselkumab in patients who showed poor response to ustekinumab.

Guselkumab is a fully monoclonal IgG1 antibody which selectively binds to the p19 subunit of IL-23. It thus prevents it from binding to the IL-23 receptor and thus preventing release of proinflammatory cytokines like IL-17A and chemokines. Ustekinumab is a human IgG1k monoclonal antibody which specifically binds to the p40 subunit protein which is used by both IL-

23 and IL-12 which are naturally occurring cytokines which are involved in immune and inflammatory responses including natural killer cell activation and CD4+ T cell differentiation and activation.

This was a double-blind randomized trial in which 871 patients were studied. All the patients received ustekinumab in a dose of 45 or 90 mg at weeks 0 and 4. At the end of 16 weeks, 268 patients had an inadequate response to ustekinumab which was having IGA (5-point Investigator's global assessment scale) of ≥2 post-treatment. These patients were randomized in a double-blind manner into two groups one of which received guselkumab in a dose of 100 mg and the rest continued ustekinumab. The patients who responded to ustekinumab (585 patients, which included those who showed inadequate response to ustekinumab in the afore mentioned) continued ustekinumab.

The two groups were compared in the following parameters; the number of visits to achieve an IGA of 0/1, at least two grade improvement from week 28 to week 40, Psoriasis Area Severity Index (PASI) 90/100 (≥ 90% or 100% improvement in PASI score) and Dermatology Life Quality Index (DLQI) of 0/1.

All the parameters studies were significantly better in the guselkumab group compared to the ustekinumab group. However, more percentage of patients had at least one adverse effect (of which the most common were infections) and one serious adverse effect in the guselkumab group compared to ustekinumab group.

This study took into consideration only patients who did not respond to ustekinumab for the randomized double-blind trial. Therefore, it is expected that the results will be in favor of guselkumab. A study which randomly allots patients into both groups without receiving either of these drugs previously is required to confirm the results of this trial. Moreover, the side effects of guselkumab also have to be taken into consideration while administering the drug.

Key Messages

- ***Guselkumab showed significantly better benefit in achieving PASI 90, PASI 100, DLQI of 0/1 and proportion of patients achieving IGA of 0/1 than ustekinumab in psoriasis patients who were not responding to ustekinumab***
- ***The adverse effects and severe adverse effects were more in guselkumab compared to ustekinumab.***

ARTICLE 44

Effect of Secukinumab on Quality of Life and Psoriasis-related Symptoms: A Comparative Analysis Versus Ustekinumab from the CLEAR 52-week Study

Puig L, Augustin M, Blauvelt A, et al. Effect of secukinumab on quality of life and psoriasis-related symptoms: A comparative analysis versus ustekinumab from the CLEAR 52-week study.
J Am Acad Dermatol. 2018;78(4):741-8.

Abstract

Secukinumab has shown better benefits than ustekinumab with respect to sustained skin clearance, improvement in symptoms, safety profile and improvement in quality of life in other studies. The objective of this study was to confirm the beneficial impact of secukinumab vs. ustekinumab with respect to cumulative benefit among patients with moderate-to-severe psoriasis, complete relief of symptoms and time to relieve psoriasis related symptoms. Data were studied from the CLEAR trial. The conclusion was that secukinumab gives greater and more sustained benefits as compared to ustekinumab in psoriasis patients.

COMMENT

This article is a comparison of secukinumab and ustekinumab on the treatment of psoriasis. The parameters considered were complete relief from psoriasis symptoms such as itching, pain and scaling, Dermatology Life Quality Index (DLQI) response, time to DLQI response, cumulative benefit in terms of reduction of Psoriasis Area Severity Index (PASI) score over a period of 52 weeks.

Secukinumab is a fully human IgG1k monoclonal antibody which selectively targets IL-17A which is a key pathogenic cytokine and has a direct action on keratinocytes to stimulate them to secrete proinflammatory mediators. Secukinumab has shown better results than ustekinumab, infliximab, adalimumab and etanercept in phase III trials at the end of 16 weeks of treatment. Secukinumab has shown better results than ustekinumab in a 52-week randomized double-blind trial. Secukinumab is given in a dose of 300 mg subcutaneously at baseline and then every week for 4 weeks and then every 4 weeks after that.

Ustekinumab is a human monoclonal antibody which is directed against cytokines IL-12 and IL-23. IL-23 activates Th17 helper cells and IL-17A and drives psoriasis pathogenesis. Ustekinumab has shown better benefit than etanercept in achieving PASI 75 response in a phase III study. Ustekinumab is given in a dose of 45 mg and 90 mg (for <100 kg and >100 kg bodyweight respectively) subcutaneously at baseline, week 4 and every 12 weeks after that.

In this study, there was a significantly better response in patients treated with secukinumab. More number of patients in the secukinumab group achieved complete relief of pain at week 16 and 32. Dermatology Life Quality Index response and cumulative response was significantly better with secukinumab.

Key Messages

- ***Secukinumab has shown to give better results than ustekinumab with respect to the time required to achieve complete remission of symptoms, DLQI response and cumulative response at the end of 52 weeks with respect to improvement of PASI score.***

ARTICLE 45

Differential Effects of Secukinumab vs. Ustekinumab for Treatment of Psoriasis on Quality of Life, Work Productivity and Activity Impairment: A Structural Equation Modelling Analysis

Stull DE, Griffiths CEM, Gilloteau I, et al. Differential effects of secukinumab vs. ustekinumab for treatment of psoriasis on quality of life, work productivity and activity impairment: A structural equation modelling analysis.
Br J Dermatol. 2018;178(6):1297-1307.

Abstract

Psoriasis has a chronic nature and this creates a significant burden on patients by causing depressive symptoms, negative self-esteem, sleep impairment and decreased work productivity. The objective of this study was to analyze the effects of ustekinumab vs. secukinumab on the work productivity, activity impairment and quality of life. CLEAR study was used for this analysis. The parameters assessed were DLQI, WPASI, PASI severity, symptoms such as itching, pain and scaling, PASI 50, 75, 90 and 100. Secukinumab gave better results in all parameters compared to ustekinumab.

COMMENT

This article is an analysis on the data from CLEAR study to compare the direct and indirect effects of secukinumab and ustekinumab. It compared the DLQI (Dermatology life quality index), WPAI (Work productivity and activity impairment)and reduction in severity, and symptoms such as itching, pain and scaling and WPAI.

The parameters were assessed at week 16 and week 52 of treatment. Number of patients achieving a Psoriasis Area Severity Index (PASI) 50, 75, 90 and 100 were taken into consideration. Analysis of patients achieving a PASI 90 was particularly analyzed.

A PASI 90 response helped to effect a change in the DLQI score as well as reduction in symptoms. Any PASI response at 16 weeks helped in getting better WPAI scores. Reduction in any of the symptoms helped to reduce WPAI.

All the parameters improved more on treatment with secukinumab than with ustekinumab.

Psoriasis has a considerable impact on the quality of life and also causes work productivity impairment. Treating the symptoms and reduction of the PASI score rapidly will help to improve the quality of life of the patient and reduce the burden of the disease on the person and the community by increasing their work productivity.

Secukinumab helps in faster reduction of these parameters than ustekinumab. Secukinumab has also been studied to be useful in patients who have been resistant to treatment with other biologics. In phase III studies, secukinumab has been found to be more useful than Tumor necrosis factor-α (TNF-α) inhibitors such as etanercept, infliximab and adalimumab.

Hence, if biologics are used in psoriasis secukinumab could be used to reduce the symptoms and signs of the disease and then followed up with other treatment modalities.

Key Messages

- ***Early reduction of the PASI score as well as the symptoms such as itching, pain and scaling helps to improve the dermatology life quality index as well as reduction of the work productivity and activity impairment scores***
- ***Secukinumab helps in better and faster reduction of the PASI scores and symptoms than ustekinumab.***

ARTICLE 46

Glucose Transporter-1 (GLUT-1) Expression in Psoriasis: Correlation with Disease Severity

Hodeib AA, Neinaa YME, Zakaria SS, et al. Glucose transporter-1 (GLUT-1) expression in psoriasis: Correlation with disease severity.
Int J Dermatol. 2018;57(8):943-51.

Abstract

Epidermal hyperproliferation along with abnormal differentiation, inflammation and angiogenesis are the key features of psoriasis. The goal of this study was to study the GLUT-1 expression in psoriasis.

The study includes 40 psoriasis vulgaris patients and 20 healthy individuals. The study evaluated the GLUT-1 level by skin biopsies taken from lesional and non-lesional skin of psoriasis patients as well as normal skin of control subjects. All biopsy specimens were examined for GLUT-1 antibody expression by immunohistochemistry and GLUT-1 mRNA expression by real-time polymerase chain reaction (RT-PCR). Besides specimens of psoriasis lesions were also stained by hematoxylin and eosin and CD31 for morphometric analysis of histopathological parameters.

Lesional skin of psoriasis patients showed more intensity of GLUT-1 immunohistochemical expression when compared to non-lesional and normal control skin. Psoriasis Area and Severity Index (PASI) score, mean of epidermal thickness, inflammatory cell density, and microvessel density have positive feedback with GLUT-1 expression in psoriasis lesions. Glucose transporter-1 could take part in a role not only in the onset of psoriasis but also in the progression and severity of the disease. It may contribute in the pathogenesis of psoriasis through the facilitation of epidermal hyperproliferation, inflammation, and angiogenesis.

COMMENT

Psoriasis is a common chronic inflammatory skin disorder. The character of this disease is excessive proliferation of keratinocytes. However, the precise mechanism of proliferation is not yet fully understood. This study highlights the role of Glucose Transporter-1 (GLUT-1) in psoriasis. It has found out that GLUT-1 could play a role not only in the onset of psoriasis, but also in the progression and severity of the disease. It may participate in the pathogenesis of psoriasis through the facilitation of epidermal hyperproliferation, inflammation, and angiogenesis.

The major source of energy for all cells is glucose. The most common glucose transporter in humans is GLUT-1. GLUT-1 is a member of facilitative sugar transporters that are integral membrane glycoproteins moving sugar across cell membrane. The study emphasizes GLUT-1 expression in psoriasis. Forty patients with psoriasis vulgaris and 20 healthy individuals were included in the study. Skin biopsies were done from lesional and non-lesional skin of psoriatic patients and normal skin of controls. All were examined for GLUT-1 antibody expression by immunohistochemistry and GLUT-1 mRNA expression by real-time polymerase chain reaction (RT-PCR).

Glucose Transporter-1 mRNA expression in psoriatic lesions were up regulated in lesional skin of psoriasis than in non-lesional and skin of controls.

Glucose Transporter-1 expression in psoriatic lesions revealed considerable positive correlations with Psoriasis Area and Severity Index (PASI) score, mean of epidermal thickness, inflammatory cell density, and microvessel density.

The study is a small study, psoriasis being a common disease it has included only 40 patients.

The study results might not match to all psoriatic patients. Future studies are required for larger population.

Key Messages

- *Glucose transporter-1 could take part not only in the onset of psoriasis, but also in the progression and severity of the disease*
- *It also contributes in the pathogenesis of psoriasis through the facilitation of epidermal hyper proliferation, inflammation, and angiogenesis.*

ARTICLE 47

Exposure to Biological Therapies during Conception and Pregnancy: A Systematic Review

Pottinger E, Woolf RT, Exton LS, et al. Exposure to biological therapies during conception and pregnancy: A systematic review.

Br J Dermatol. 2018;178(1):95-102.

Abstract

Nowadays biological therapies are also added in the treatment list of psoriatic females during pregnancy and conception.

Pregnant women treated with TNF-α blockers three months prior and after conception of pregnancy are taken into account.

Preterm birth and congenital anomalies are noted in very few patients which even doesn't have a statistical importance.

Pregnant women when are in need to use biologics the benefit risk ratio should be overweighed.

COMMENT

Psoriasis mainly of its complete incurable nature, diverse clinical features stay as a social stigma more in females of reproductive age group. That's why even biologics are added up in the treatment ladder of female patient in pregnancy.

Tumor necrosis factor (TNF) α-blockers treated patients in pregnancy and three months prior to conception are considered. Congenital anomalies and premature birth are evident in very few pregnant women. However, statistical importance of adverse effect is not evident.

The exact mechanism of TNF-α blockers in embryogenesis is not known clearly. The embryo, entire female reproductive tract and even the placenta are found to have TNF-α in tissues. It has been postulated that TNF-α plays a role in defense mechanism of embryo. Thus in theory TNF-α blocker may affect the embryogenesis.

The article has taken biologics used for all diseases. More studies are warranted for psoriatic population of reproductive age.

Use of biologicals in pregnant patient should be decided individually among each patient. Benefit should be carefully overweighed among risk in patient who are going to conceive or in pregnant women.

Key Messages

- ***Major congenital malformations were reported in less than 5% of women exposed to TNFi during the first trimester***
- ***When planning conception the risks and benefits of continuing vs. stopping therapy should be planned on a case-by-case basis.***

ARTICLE 48

Higher Coronary Plaque Burden in Psoriatic Arthritis is Independent of Metabolic Syndrome and Associated with Underlying Disease Severity

Szentpetery A, Healy GM, Brady D, et al. Higher coronary plaque burden in psoriatic arthritis is independent of metabolic syndrome and associated with underlying disease severity.
Arthritis Rheumatol. 2018;70(3):396-407.

Abstract

The study is conducted in psoriatic arthritis (PsA) patients. It is to scrutinize the effect of metabolic syndrome and coronary plaque burden; 64-slice coronary computed tomography angiography was done in 50 PsA patients without coronary artery disease (CAD). A total of 50 age- and sex-matched controls were added in the study. The factors examined are plaque localization, segment involvement score (SIS), segment stenosis score (SSS), and total plaque volume (TPV) .The study found that plaques in 76% of PsA patients versus 44% of controls ($p = 0.001$). The independent predictors of higher plaque burden in PsA are age, highest C-reactive protein level, highest swollen joint count and disease duration; coronary plaque formation, particularly mixed plaques is seen in PsA.

COMMENT

Psoriasis (Ps) and psoriatic arthritis (PsA) belong to the family of immune mediated inflammatory diseases (IMID), affecting predominantly the skin and joints. The prevalence of Ps varies between 2% and 3% worldwide with a similar distribution among male and female. It has been estimated that 7–42% of Ps patients develop an inflammatory arthropathy, usually manifesting as a mono or asymmetrical oligoarthritis. Substantial body of evidence suggests that PsA patients are at higher risk of developing atherosclerotic cardiovascular disease

Psoriasis has a bimodal distribution of incidence, with a first peak in patients between 20 and 30 years old and a second peak in patients 50–60 years of age. Because this second peak coincides with the age range that patients are also more likely to develop overt coronary artery disease (CAD), recognizing the increased risk of CAD in older patients with incident Ps may have important implications for preventing future cardiovascular events.

Psoriasis may be an independent risk factor for premature cardiovascular disease. A small number of studies have found the association between the risk of cardiovascular morbidity and Ps severity. They also have demonstrated an augmented risk of peripheral vascular disease, stroke, and mortality in Ps patients.

The article has found out that patients with well-established PsA without any symptoms or a diagnosis of coronary artery disease have a higher burden of coronary plaques, which may be linked to underlying disease activity and severity, but is independent of features of metabolic syndrome.

To assess the coronary plaque burden the participants underwent 64-slice coronary computed tomography angiography. Examiners calculated plaque localization, segment stenosis score, segment involvement score, and total plaque volume.

Patients with and without metabolic syndrome had similar plaque burdens and types of plaques. Segment stenosis score, segment involvement score, and total plaque volume were significantly associated with features of disease activity.

It was concluded that PsA is linked with accelerated plaque formation, mainly mixed plaques, which is independent of the presence of metabolic syndrome.

Key Message

- ***PsA is linked with accelerated plaque formation, mainly mixed plaques, which is independent of the presence of metabolic syndrome.***

ARTICLE 49

Increased Levels of Lipocalin 2 in Palmoplantar Pustular Psoriasis

Wolk K, Frambach Y, Jacobi A, et al. Increased levels of lipocalin 2 in palmoplantar pustular psoriasis. *J Dermatol Sci. 2018;90(1):68-74.*

Abstract

The study was conducted to determine and characterize pathogenetic players in palmoplantar pustular psoriasis (PPP).

The study collected clinical data and blood samples of 60 PPP patients. Healthy individuals were served as controls.

In PPP patients, lipocalin 2 (LCN2) found to be significantly up regulated compared to healthy participants. Lipocalin 2 was produced by keratinocytes in PPP skin lesions. *In vitro,* LCN2 production of these cells was influenced by IL-1β and further improved by IL-17 and TNF-α, while IL-22 had no effect. In PPP increased LCN2 denotes a vital activity of IL-1β in the epidermis, and this may add to skin neutrophil infiltration and pro-atherosclerosis risk.

COMMENT

Palmoplantar pustular psoriasis (PPP) is a variant of psoriasis affecting the palms and soles. Palmoplantar pustulosis occurs as crops of sterile pustules on one or both hands and/or feet. They also develop red scaly plaque with deep fissures.

Palmoplantar pustulosis has exacerbations and remissions. The distress can be substantial, interfering with work and leisure activities. The etiology of palmoplantar pustulosis is not completely understood. Palmoplantar pustular psoriasis is an autoimmune disease, in the sense that the immune defenses of the body acts against itself. This study tries to make out and typify pathogenetic players in PPP.

Along with clinical data skin and blood samples of 60 PPP patients were collected. Healthy participants were used as controls. Enzyme-linked immunosorbent assay (ELISA), quantitative Real-time polymerase chain reaction (qRT-PCR), and immunohistochemistry were done for analysis of patient samples and cultured primary skin cells.

Lipocalin-2 (LCN2), also called as oncogene 24p3 or neutrophil gelatinase-associated lipocalin (NGAL), is a protein present in humans. Neutrophils expressed it. On screening of blood levels in PPP patients, LCN2 emerged as being appreciably increased compared to healthy participants.

Interleukin (IL)-1β up regulates LCN2 production. IL-17 further improves the production. PPP show a positive relationship between blood IL-1β and LCN2 levels. Vital activity of IL-1β in the epidermis is by increased LCN2 in PPP. This is responsible for skin neutrophil accumulation and pro-atherosclerosis risk.

Key Message

- ***In PPP, increased blood levels of LCN2 point to an important activity of IL-1β in the epidermis, may add to skin neutrophil infiltration.***

ARTICLE 50

Ixekizumab Treatment for Psoriasis: Integrated Efficacy Analysis of Three Double-blinded, Controlled Studies (UNCOVER-1, UNCOVER-2, UNCOVER-3)

Papp KA, Leonardi CL, Blauvelt A, et al. Ixekizumab treatment for psoriasis: Integrated efficacy analysis of three double-blinded, controlled studies (UNCOVER-1, UNCOVER-2, UNCOVER-3).
Br J Dermatol. 2018;178(3):674-81.

Abstract

The article analyze efficacy of ixekizumab in psoriasis from three studies (UNCOVER-1, UNCOVER-2, UNCOVER-3). Data are collected for induction period.

Ixekizumab (IXE) treatment was better to placebo ($p<0.001$) and etanercept ($p<0.001$) on sPGA (0, 1) and PASI 75, with noteworthy differences in PASI improvement at week 1. Ixekizumab Q2W was higher to IXE Q4W on all treatment outcomes.

At both dosing regimens ixekizumab therapy showed rapid onset and greater efficacy to placebo and etanercept, with IXE Q2W giving better outcomes than IXE Q4W during the first 12 weeks of treatment.

COMMENT

Psoriasis is a chronic, relapsing immune-mediated inflammatory skin disorder. The plaque-type psoriasis (psoriasis vulgaris) is characterized by erythematous, well-circumscribed papules and plaques covered with silvery scales on extensor surfaces and other cutaneous locations.

Interleukin (IL)-23 and IL-17 are central in the pathogenesis of plaque psoriasis. Various biologics are targeted against them. Anti-IL-17 biologics are brodalumab, secukinumab and ixekizumab (IXE).

A humanized monoclonal antibody that inhibits the IL-17 is ixekizumab and it is approved by FDA for psoriatic patients. Three major phase III trials, UNCOVER-1, UNCOVER-2, and UNCOVER-3, were conducted to evaluate the efficacy, safety, and impact on quality of life of this new agent. Three pivotal phase III studies have assessed the efficacy of IXE dose regimens compared with placebo (PBO), and two of the studies included the active comparator etanercept (ETN).

The study hypothesized that IXE would provide highly effective therapy for patients with moderate-to-severe plaque psoriasis that is superior to PBO and to ETN. In addition, the study also hypothesized that the response to IXE 80 mg every 2 weeks (Q2W) would be greater than the response to IXE 80 every 4 weeks (Q4W) across all efficacy measures.

Ixekizumab demonstrated statistically significant separation from PBO and ETN as early as week 1 in mean improvement in Psoriasis Area Severity Index (PASI) score. Ixekizumab at the most efficacious dosing (Q2W), achieves the highest PASI 75 of all IL-17 and IL-23 axis agents. Events reported at a significantly greater frequency in the total IXE group compared with PBO were non specified injection-site reaction (ISR), injection-site erythema, and nausea and oropharyngeal pain.

The integrated analysis reported here replicates the rapid onset and the superiority of IXE treatment over ETN or PBO. The majority of patients achieved minimal disease severity, with approximately 40% achieving complete resolution of psoriasis after 12 weeks of IXE Q2W treatment. Patients treated with the IXE Q2W dosing regimen had significantly better treatment outcomes than those treated with IXE Q4W.

Key Messages

- ***Ixekizumab at the most efficacious dosing (Q2W), achieves the highest PASI 75 of all IL-17 and IL-23 axis agents***
- ***Patients treated with the IXE Q2W dosing regimen had significantly better treatment outcomes than those treated with IXE Q4W.***

ARTICLE 51

Long-term Clinical Efficacy and Safety of Secukinumab for Japanese Patients with Psoriasis: A Single-center Experience

Momose M, Asahina A, Umezawa Y, et al. Long-term clinical efficacy and safety of secukinumab for Japanese patients with psoriasis: A single-center experience.
J Dermatol. 2018;45(3):318-21.

Abstract

This study describe the long-term clinical efficacy and safety of secukinumab for Japanese psoriatic patients with psoriasis in a single-center. Secukinumab showed significant Psoriasis Area and Severity Index (PASI) 75 and PASI 90 responses. No remarkable differences were observed in efficacy between bio-naive and bio-switched patients. Secukinumab for PsA improved arthralgia by week 12 with a reduction of serum C-reactive protein level. In Japanese psoriatic patients secukinumab showed a constant clinical response with a satisfactory safety profile.

COMMENT

Psoriasis is a chronic, immune-mediated, inflammatory skin disease and is characterized by inflammatory cell infiltration, epidermal cell hyperproliferation and dilated microvessels. The disease is frequently associated with other chronic and serious health conditions such as metabolic syndromes and cardiovascular disorders. Furthermore, psoriasis causes considerable psychosocial disability, thereby exerting substantial burden on the daily life of patients.

The study was a retrospective study which analyzed psoriasis and psoriatic arthritis treated with secukinumab between May 2015 and August 2016. The incidence of psoriasis in males was more than twice as high as that in females. Psoriasis reportedly occurs predominantly in males in Japan, unlike Western countries where the male: female ratio is equal.

Interleukin (IL)-23 and IL-17 are central in the pathogenesis of plaque psoriasis. Novel biologic agents are targeted against them. Anti-IL-17 biologics are brodalumab, secukinumab and ixekizumab.

Secukinumab is a recombinant, fully human immunoglobulin G1 kappa monoclonal antibody that selectively binds to interleukin (IL)-17A and neutralizes its bioactivity. Secukinumab was used for psoriasis, psoriatic arthritis (PsA) and pustular psoriasis in Japan (2014). It showed excellent efficacy compared to placebo, etanercept or ustekinumab.

Secukinumab Japanese patients showed Psoriasis Area Severity Index (PASI) 75 and PASI 90 in more than 80% and 60% respectively.

Secukinumab showed remarkable improvement in PsA by relieving their joint pain and lesser C-reactive protein (CRP) levels. Tumor necrosis factor (TNF)-α inhibitors rank top in treating PsA patients, however in special circumstances, secukinumab also used for PsA.

Secukinumab effectiveness was sustained for 52 weeks. The small sample size is the limitation of this study.

Key Messages

- *Japanese psoriatic patients showed PASI 75 in more than 80% in Secukinumab treated patients*
- *Secukinumab effectiveness was sustained for 52 weeks.*

ARTICLE 52

Matching-adjusted Indirect Comparison of Efficacy in Patients with Moderate-to-Severe Plaque Psoriasis Treated with Ixekizumab vs. Secukinumab

Warren RB, Brnabic A, Saure D, et al. Matching-adjusted indirect comparison of efficacy in patients with moderate-to-severe plaque psoriasis treated with ixekizumab vs. secukinumab.
Br J Dermatol. 2018;178(5):1064-71.

Abstract

The study assess efficacy of ixekizumab and secukinumab in psoriatic patients using matching-adjusted indirect comparisons.

Dermatology Life Quality Index (DLQI) and Psoriasis Area and Severity Index (PASI) of patients treated with ixekizumab and secukinumab were compared. Bucher (BU) method and two modified versions of the Signorovitch (SG) method (SG total and SG separate) were used for comparisons.

At week 12 ixekizumab showed higher PASI 90 and PASI 100 responses compared with secukinumab.

COMMENT

Psoriasis is a chronic, relapsing immune-mediated inflammatory skin disorder. Despite recent advancements, the immunopathogenesis of psoriasis remains incompletely understood. Basically, psoriasis is a T-helper (Th) 1 driven disease.

Biologics have topped the treatment ladder in psoriasis. This is because of rapid visible clearance and nil organ damage.

The study compared the effectiveness and life quality of psoriatic patients treated with two main biologics like ixekizumab versus secukinumab. It is an indirect comparison.

Signorovitch comparison method was less biased. It compares ixekizumab and secukinumab by adjusting the baseline clinical differences. Ixekizumab showed a good Psoriasis Area Severity Index (PASI) response. The rate of action was faster in ixekizumab treated patients.

The pitfalls of the study are it failed to analyze the adverse effects, as many adverse effects are very rare.

Signorovitch comparison method is a boon to the research field as it is less biased. The advantage of this study is it compares with other biologics.

Ixekizumab showed a very good response compared to secukinumab. Psoriasis Area Severity Index clearance was rapid in ixekizumab.

Key Messages

- ***Ixekizumab had higher PASI 90 and PASI 100 responses at week 12 compared with secukinumab using adjusted indirect comparisons***
- ***Ixekizumab has more rapid onset of action.***

ARTICLE 53

Metabolic Syndrome in Psoriatic Arthritis: The Interplay with Cutaneous Involvement. Evidences from Literature and a Recent Cross-sectional Study

Caso F, Del Puente A, Oliviero F, et al. Metabolic syndrome in psoriatic arthritis: The interplay with cutaneous involvement. Evidences from literature and a recent cross-sectional study.
Clin Rheumatol. 2018;37(3):579-86.

Abstract

The cross-sectional study evaluates the serum uric acid and occurrence of metabolic syndrome (MetS) in PsA patients and in those with PsA sine psoriasis. Additionally the study investigated on MetS correlations in all study population. Glucose, lipid profile, serum uric acid, and acute-phase reactants were analyzed from blood samples. In psoriasis, increase of one unit of BMI and smoking habit reached statistical significance: PsA patients have more occurrence of MetS and higher levels of serum uric acid compared to PsA sine psoriasis. Body mass index, psoriasis, and smoking are key determinants in the development of MetS in PsA patients.

COMMENT

Psoriasis (PsO) is a T cell (Th1 and Th17)-mediated chronic inflammatory skin disorder with clinically apparent joint involvement in nearly 30% of patients. Neema Ali et al. reported prevalence of psoriatic arthritis (PsA) varies from 1 to 420 cases (median 180) per 10^5 population and affects men and women equally. Obesity, dyslipidemia, hyperglycemia and hypertension together constitutes metabolic syndrome (MetS). It is one of the major global health issues. Multiple studies in India and abroad conducted over the past few years have confirmed the increased prevalence of MetS in psoriatic patients when compared with normal healthy controls. This is because PsO is a prototypical Th1 inflammatory disease characterized by expansion and activation of Th1 T cells, antigen-presenting cells and Th1 cytokines. Similarly, chronic Th1 inflammation is important to the pathophysiology of obesity, MetS, diabetes, atherosclerosis and myocardial infarction.

The aim of this study was to assess the prevalence of MetS and its components and the level of serum uric acid in patients with PsA and in those with PsA sine psoriasis. A secondary aim of the study was to scrutinize on correlations of MetS in all study population.

The study demonstrated that MetS was more in PsA with PsO than PsA sine PsO. The higher prevalence of MetS in PsA was consistent with the findings of Pehlevan et al. and Raychaudhuri et al. This is in contrast to that of Bostoen et al. which showed a decreased prevalence of MetS in PsA patients than in PsO patients.

Psoriatic arthritis patients should always be monitored for cardiovascular events. As truncal obesity and dyslipidemia were the most common components of MetS in PsA, lifestyle modification, diet changes and weight reduction may go a long way in reducing the incidence of MetS in patients with PsA. A drawback of this study is the small sample size.

Key Messages

- ***The study demonstrates that MetS was more in PsA with psoriasis than PsA sine psoriasis***
- ***The study also show the potential role of BMI, psoriasis, and smoking as important determinants in the development of MetS in PsA patients.***

ARTICLE 54

IL-17C: A Unique Epithelial Cytokine with Potential for Targeting across the Spectrum of Atopic Dermatitis and Psoriasis

Guttman-Yassky E, Krueger JG. IL-17C: A unique epithelial cytokine with potential for targeting across the spectrum of atopic dermatitis and psoriasis.
J Invest Dermatol. 2018;138(7):1467-9.

Abstract

Complex inflammatory circuits regulated by "feed-forward" mechanisms are seen in both atopic dermatitis (AD) and psoriasis. Keratinocyte-derived cytokines and inflammatory mediators amplify cellular immune responses. Unique cytokine namely IL-17C is involved in synergistic loops responsible for amplifying the inflammation in two diseases. The ultimate result is the induction of S100As that accompany epidermal hyperplasia. Thus, opposition of IL-17C will be beneficial in both psoriasis and AD patients. The therapeutic possibility of IL-17C antagonism in AD is evidenced by a recently reported small phase 1 clinical trial in patients with AD.

COMMENT

Atopic dermatitis (AD) and psoriasis are polar immune diseases. Basically, AD is a T helper 2 (Th2) and psoriasis T helper 1 (Th1) driven disease. This article states that AD also has variable Th1 and Th17 activation. The complex inflammatory circuits in both diseases are regulated through feed forward mechanism which amplifies the immune and inflammatory responses.

Keratinocytes primarily produces IL-17C. It is involved in synergistic loops responsible for amplifying the inflammation. AD and psoriasis shows higher IL-17C expression. IL-17C participates in both autocrine signaling in the epidermis and paracrine signaling to immune cells. There is also strong synergy between IL-17C and NF-κB (nuclear factor kappa-light-chain-enhancer of activated B cells) activators, such as IL-1 or Tumor necrosis factor (TNF), and a synergy with IL-22 has also been reported. This may ultimately lead to induction of S100A7-9 molecules that are proteins responsible for cellular differentiation and psoriasiform hyperplasia in both conditions.

Atopic dermatitis patients respond well to IL-17 antagonist showing 50% improvement in severity score. Patient showed improvement for next 8 weeks.

Limitation of the study is small sample size. Future studies are warranted for larger population to represent the general population.

Key Messages

- *Atopic dermatitis, Th2 mediated has variable Th1/Th17 activation*
- *The IL-17C neutralizing antibody MOR 106 was able to inhibit both T helper type 2 cells and T helper type 17/T helper type 22-skewed inflammatory loops that drive different features of AD and psoriasis.*

ARTICLE 55

Patient-reported Symptoms and Signs of Moderate-to-Severe Psoriasis Treated with Guselkumab or Adalimumab: Results from the Randomized VOYAGE 1 trial

Papp KA, Blauvelt A, Kimball AB, et al. Patient-reported symptoms and signs of moderate-to-severe psoriasis treated with guselkumab or adalimumab: Results from the randomized VOYAGE 1 trial.
J Eur Acad Dermatol Venereol. 2018;32(9):1515-22.

Abstract

The article assesses patient-reported symptoms and signs of moderate-to-severe psoriasis treated with guselkumab or adalimumab from a randomized VOYAGE 1 trial.

The proportion of patients attaining clinically significant improvements in PSSD summary scores was appreciably higher in the guselkumab group compared with the placebo group at week 16 and compared with the adalimumab group at weeks 24 and 48.

Guselkumab showed greater improvements in symptoms and signs of psoriasis based on PSSD scores than adalimumab and placebo.

COMMENT

Quality of life is very much affected in psoriatic patients. Morphology of psoriatic lesions is considered as stigma. Psoriasis of scalp and nail are cumbersome to treat. Biologics are used in the treatment of psoriasis in the last decade.

The article assesses the patient reported psoriatic symptoms and signs of biologics like adalimumab, a tumor necrosis factor-α (TNF-α) inhibitor and guselkumab, blocker of interleukin 23 (IL-23). The article is based on studies conducted globally for two years.

Records of psoriatic signs and symptoms of patient are used. Itching, pain and tightening of skin are taken into account. Inflammation, pinpoint bleeding and shedding of scales are evaluated.

Based on patient record, guselkumab given for psoriasis showed rapid onset of action. Treatment resistant areas also respond to guselkumab. Guselkumab treated patients give a visible clearance compare to its competitor biologics at an earlier week.

Guselkumab is superior to adalimumab in treating psoriasis. Safety profile is also more for guselkumab. In the psoriasis pathogenesis, IL-23 play a vital role compared to TNF-α inhibitor.

Key Message

- ***Guselkumab was superior in showing a visible clearance at an earlier week.***

ARTICLE 56

Effects of Treatment for Psoriasis on Circulating Levels of Leptin, Adiponectin and Resistin: A Systematic Review and Meta-analysis

Kyriakou A, Patsatsi A, Sotiriadis D, et al. Effects of treatment for psoriasis on circulating levels of leptin, adiponectin and resistin: A systematic review and meta-analysis.
Br J Dermatol. 2018;179(2):273-81.

Abstract

The study is a systematic review and meta-analysis to find the effects of treatment for psoriasis on circulating levels of leptin, adiponectin and resistin. Metabolic syndrome is more common in psoriatic patients than in the general population. Circulating adipokine levels are altered in patients with psoriasis. It suggests a pathophysiological link between psoriatic lesions and metabolic alterations.

Three databases (PubMed, Central and Embase) were used for search. Studies that assessed leptin, adiponectin or resistin concentrations were taken into consideration.

There is no proof that treatment for psoriasis alters leptin and adiponectin levels. However, treatment intervention lowers resistin concentrations, a finding that is estimated to be of clinical importance.

COMMENT

Psoriasis is an immune-mediated, inflammatory disease. Psoriasis can lead to substantial morbidity and mortality directly from the disease as well as from the effect of comorbidities. Metabolic syndrome, a risk factor of cardiovascular disease, is more common in patients with psoriasis than in the general population. Adipokine contribute to the regulation of immune-mediated processes and inflammation. List of adipokines secreted by adipose tissue that are considered as possible markers of metabolic syndrome are leptin, adiponectin, and resistin.

This is a review article that evaluated the circulating concentrations of adipokine in patients with psoriasis and controls and has meta-analyzed the best evidence available. The article has assessed leptin, resistin, or adiponectin concentrations in psoriatic patients and a reference group. The study was conducted in adherence with the PRISMA (Preferred Reporting Items for Systematic Reviews and Meta-Analyses) standards.

The article has found out that leptin and adiponectin levels remain unaltered after treatment in psoriatic patients. Whereas resistin levels has lowered down after psoriasis treatment. Resistin is a 12.5 kDa polypeptide that belongs to the inflammatory zone protein family. Resistin regulates insulin sensitivity and glucose metabolism, and is a mediator between diabetes and obesity exhibiting a positive correlation with body mass index importantly, resistin induces the secretion of pro-inflammatory cytokines, such as interleukin-6 (IL-6), IL-12 and tumor necrosis factor-α (TNF-α). Interestingly, high serum resistin levels are also observed in psoriasis patients directly affect the pathogenesis of psoriasis. Resistin might be a possible biomarker for diagnosis and prognosis in psoriatic patients.

The article suggested pathogenic link between psoriasis and metabolic syndrome/ obesity is reinforced and the role of co morbidities in psoriasis is highlighted.

The limitation inherent to all meta-analysis is the possibility of publication bias, which results from publication of studies with favorable results, which is much easier than publication of unfavorable results. Another potential limitation is this analysis was conducted on psoriasis patients differing in clinical severity and receiving various treatments, all of which could have an influence on the results. Despite the above limitations, the article has highlighted the association between serum resistin levels and psoriasis. Treatment for psoriasis did not appear to modify leptin and adiponectin concentrations. In contrast, treatment intervention reduced resistin concentrations.

Key Messages

- *Resistin is a potential biomarker for diagnosis and prognosis in psoriatic patients*
- *Treatment for psoriasis did not appear to modify leptin and adiponectin concentrations. In contrast, treatment intervention reduced resistin concentrations*
- *Resistin is a 12.5 kDa polypeptide that belongs to the inflammatory zone protein family.*

ARTICLE 57

Subcutaneous Methotrexate in Patients with Moderate-to-Severe Psoriasis: A Critical Appraisal

Tsakok T, Jabbar-Lopez ZK, Smith CH. Subcutaneous methotrexate in patients with moderate-to-severe psoriasis: A critical appraisal.
Br J Dermatol. 2018;179(1):50-53.

Abstract

This study assessed the use of an intense dose schedule of subcutaneous methotrexate in patients having moderate-to-severe plaque psoriasis. Patients with moderate-to-severe plaque psoriasis who were not treated with methotrexate were given subcutaneous methotrexate or a placebo both for a duration of 16 weeks in the first phase of this study. This was followed by both the groups receiving methotrexate injections once a week. This 52-week study conducted with 120 patients proved a good risk benefit profile of giving subcutaneous methotrexate.

COMMENT

Methotrexate is one of the most commonly used drugs used for the treatment of psoriasis. It is also a cost-effective option and even after the patients are treated with other agents like biologics or cyclosporine, methotrexate is commonly given for a long duration of time after tapering and stoppage of other medications.

The dose which is usually given in Indian patients is 5 mg to 15 mg per week usually in an oral mode of administration either in single weekly dose or in divided doses. In this study, a dose of 17.5 mg and if not responding a dose of 22.5 mg per week administered subcutaneously was given. This study was done with 120 patients which was a randomized double-blind prospective study done in 16 centers of four countries.

Chronic plaque psoriasis patients who were methotrexate naïve were divided into two groups. One group was given methotrexate subcutaneously in a dose of 17.5 mg once a week increased to 22.5 mg once weekly if there was no Psoriasis Area Severity Index (PASI) 50 response by the 8th week. The other group was treated with a placebo. The patients were given folic acid 5 mg per week. After 16 weeks, in the second phase of the study, both groups were treated with methotrexate. A dose escalation of 22.5 mg per week was given in patients who did not achieve PASI 50 at week 24. The results were measured using PASI score along with two other psoriasis severity scores and two life quality scores. Biopsies were also performed at baseline at week 16. Immunohistochemistry, interleukin, interferon and histopathology were studied. The main outcome studied was the proportion of patients achieving PASI 75 at week 16. There were no serious side effects associated with this treatment during the duration of this study.

Key Message

- ***An intense dose of subcutaneous methotrexate was effective and showed a significant risk benefit ratio in treating patients with chronic plaque psoriasis over a period of 52 weeks.***

ARTICLE 58

Management of Psoriasis in Patients with Inflammatory Bowel Disease: From the Medical Board of the National Psoriasis Foundation

Whitlock SM, Enos CW, Armstrong AW, et al. Management of psoriasis in patients with inflammatory bowel disease: From the Medical Board of the National Psoriasis Foundation.
J Am Acad Dermatol. 2018;78(2):383-94.

Abstract

The association between inflammatory bowel disease (IBD) and psoriasis is significant. There are some common treatment modalities for these two disorders. The objective of this study was to find out the optimal treatment options for patients having IBD and psoriasis. A literature search and analysis was done for the medications used in psoriasis and IBD. Adalimumab and infliximab showed significant efficacy in patients with IBD and psoriasis.

COMMENT

Psoriasis and inflammatory bowel disease (IBD) have been known to have a significant association. There are common modalities of treatment for both disorders. The therapeutic modalities for patients having both psoriasis and IBD were assessed in this study. A literature search was conducted for studies using biologics and other systemic medications in IBD such as ulcerative colitis and Crohn's disease as well as psoriasis and psoriatic arthritis (PsA) for a period of 1 month. The highest evidence-based studies i.e., randomized double-blind trails were the most preferred studies followed by the other evidence-based studies. Over 2,000 articles were obtained out of which 132 served the purpose of this analysis. The two drugs which were effective in all four disorders were two tumor necrosis factor inhibitors (TNFi) adalimumab and infliximab and therefore these should be preferred. Ustekinumab showed benefit in three of the conditions exception being ulcerative colitis. Crohn's disease and PsA showed response to certolizumab. Drugs like ixekizumab, secukinumab, brodalumab and etanercept showed benefit in PsA and psoriasis, but induced or exacerbated IBD. These are all results based on these drugs being used separately for the respective conditions. There need to be clinical trials on patients having both IBD and psoriasis to confirm these findings.

Key Message

- *Adalimumab and infliximab have shown benefit in Crohn's disease, ulcerative colitis, psoriasis as well as psoriatic arthritis. Hence, these two agents are to be preferred in patients having concurrent IBD and psoriasis.*

ARTICLE 59

Interleukin 17, Inflammation, and Cardiovascular Risk in Patients with Psoriasis

Lockshin B, Balgula Y, Merola JF. Interleukin 17, inflammation, and cardiovascular risk in patients with psoriasis. *J Am Acad Dermatol. 2018;79(2):345-52.*

Abstract

Psoriasis is a chronic inflammatory condition which apart from cutaneous involvement also has systemic manifestations. Patients who have an early onset of the disease and more severe disease have increased incidence of comorbidities and decreased life expectancy. Cardiovascular disease is one of the comorbidities of psoriasis and it is the most common etiology of mortality and morbidity in psoriatic individuals. Interleukin-17 inflammation is known to of pathogenetic importance in both cardiovascular disease and psoriasis. In this article, the association between these two conditions as well as the education and management of patients with respect to these two conditions will be discussed.

COMMENT

Psoriasis is known to be associated with cardiovascular disease (CVD). Early markers of subclinical atherosclerosis are also known to be associated with psoriasis even prior to occurrence of a cardiovascular event. Moreover, decrease in psoriasis severity has also been associated with decreases in inflammation of the vasculature.

The pathogenesis of psoriasis has involvement of many inflammatory mediators such as interleukin (IL)-17A, 17F, 22, 23, 6, 12, 1β, interferon (IFN)-γ and IFN-α. These mediators are secreted from Th1, Th17 cells as well as dendritic cells, keratinocytes and other T cells. There are various common pathogenic mechanisms in psoriasis and CVD such as inflammatory markers, chemo and cytokine profiles and systemic, and local immunologic processes. Psoriasis is also associated with obesity and adipokines cause CVD, and metabolic syndrome. In this review, the role of IL-17 in relation to CVD and psoriasis is discussed.

Interleukin-17 and 23 are secreted by Th17 cells which cause intralesional angiogenesis and keratinocyte proliferation. Thl cells cause growth of atherosclerotic plaque and intraplaque hemorrhage and neoangiogenesis is promoted by Th17 cells. Increase in the levels of intraplaque Th17 cells causes fibrous cap weakening which further leads to rupture of the plaque and myocardial infarction.

The recurrence rate of stroke, myocardial infraction and death resulting from cardiovascular events is significantly more in patients with psoriasis compared to those without psoriasis. This risk also increases with severity of psoriasis.

Both patients with psoriasis and with CVD have increase in the number of circulating Th17 cells and associated cytokines such as IL-17A.

Medications having anti-inflammatory effects proximal to IL-17A include tumor necrosis factor inhibitors (TNFi) and methotrexate. Certain studies have shown that systemic anti-inflammatory treatment of psoriasis reduced the risk of CVD and prevents recurrence of cardiovascular events.

The use of IL-17A inhibitors such as secukinumab is being studied in a group of 3,420 patients. The occurrence of cardiovascular events in patients treated with secukinumab was similar to those treated with etanercept in spite of the secukinumab group having more risk factors of CVD prior to treatment.

Appropriate screening and evaluation of patients with psoriasis for CVD risk factors should be done and it should be managed and the patients were counseled to prevent the risk of occurrence of cardiovascular events and to decrease the morbidity of the disease.

Further studies with IL-17 antagonists need to be done in patients with psoriasis and risk of CVD.

Key Messages

- ***Psoriasis is a chronic inflammatory disease having systemic apart from cutaneous manifestations and is known to be associated with cardiovascular disease***
- ***There is a similarity in pathogenetic mechanisms between psoriasis and CVD especially involving Th17 and IL-17A***
- ***The use of systemic anti-inflammatory medications such as methotrexate and TNFi are known to also reduce the risk and recurrence rate of CVD***
- ***More studies are warranted on the use of IL-17A antagonists such as secukinumab to prove a beneficial role in CVD associated with psoriasis.***

ARTICLE 60

Levels of miR-31 and its Target Genes in Dermal Mesenchymal Cells of Patients with Psoriasis

Wang Q, Chang W, Yang X, et al. Levels of miR-31 and its target genes in dermal mesenchymal cells of patients with psoriasis.
Int J Dermatol. 2018;doi:10.1111/ijd.14197.

Abstract

Psoriasis is a chronic inflammatory disease and its pathogenesis is thought to be related with dysregulation of miR-31 expression and mesenchymal stem cells (MSCs). The aim of this study was to identify the role of miR-31 in dermal MSCs in psoriasis pathogenesis.

COMMENT

In this study, miR-31 expression was studied by means of a microarray and quantitative polymerase chain reaction (PCR) was used to assess the miR-31 target genes. A control group of patients without psoriasis was also studied.

It was found that the expression of miR-31 in the psoriasis group was significantly lower than in the control group. There was four to five-fold increased expression of *EIG121L* and *EMP1* genes (whose effects are seen on the cell membrane) in psoriatic individuals compared to the control group. There was 1.1 to 7-fold increase in expression of genes expressing in the cytoplasm such as *TACC2, RNF144B, QKI, PTPN14* and *GRB10*. The expression of genes whose products play a role in the nucleus and of those whose products are seen in the extracellular space were also increased in the psoriatic patients.

This increase in expression of target genes may be attributed to the decreased expression of miR-31 in patients of psoriasis. This increased expression of target genes may lead to inhibition in proliferation of dermal mesenchymal stem cells which can lead to T-lymphocyte activation in psoriatic individuals.

This study provides another cause of pathogenesis of psoriasis apart from those already known.

Key Message

- ***There is decreased expression in miR-31 in psoriatic patients which leads to increased expression of genes with products in the cell membrane, cytoplasm, nucleus and extracellular space. This in turn leads to decreased proliferation of dermal mesenchymal stem cells which results in T-lymphocyte activation.***

ARTICLE 61

Serum Elafin as a Potential Inflammatory Marker in Psoriasis

Elgharib I, Khashaba SA, Elsaid HH, et al. Serum elafin as a potential inflammatory marker in psoriasis. ***Int J Dermatol. 2018. doi: 10.1111/ijd.14217.***

Abstract

There are various pathogenic mechanisms interplaying in the occurrence of psoriasis. This study's aim was to compare the serum elafin levels in cases of psoriasis and controls. It also compared the elafin levels with the severity of psoriasis as well as with other inflammatory markers such as ESR and CRP.

COMMENT

Psoriasis is a chronic inflammatory disorder with systemic as well as local inflammation. Therefore, elevation of serum inflammatory markers is expected in psoriasis.

Elafin is an inflammatory marker and is also known as skin derived antileukoprotease and peptidase inhibitor 3. It is a protein encoded by *PI3* gene. Elafin is known to be used as a biomarker in graft versus host disease and also has a role in gut inflammation.

In this case-control study, 26 patients with psoriasis with an equal number of controls were studied. Enzyme-linked immunosorbent assay (ELISA) was used to determine the serum elafin levels in both cases and controls. The Psoriasis Area Severity Index (PASI) score, erythrocyte sedimentation rate (ESR) and C-reactive protein (CRP) were done in the psoriasis cases.

There were statistically significant higher levels of elafin in the psoriasis patients compared to controls. The p-value was <0.001 which indicates a high level of significance. The severity of psoriasis (determined by the PASI score) also showed a significant correlation with elafin levels. Further, there was a correlation between the CRP and ESR which are also markers of inflammation and the elafin levels.

Therefore, elafin can be used as a marker for the severity of psoriasis. It can be especially useful in case of systemic inflammation where cutaneous findings may not be that severe. Further studies with a larger number of subjects and randomization and blinding are necessary to prove the role of elafin in the prognosis of psoriasis.

Key Message

- ***Elafin levels are significantly elevated in psoriasis patients compared to controls and it also correlated with the severity of psoriasis as well as with other inflammatory markers such as CRP and ESR.***

ARTICLE 62

Sex Hormones, Erectile Dysfunction, and Psoriasis; A Bad Friendship!

Eltaweel AEAI, Mustafa AI, El-Shimi OS, et al. Sex hormones, erectile dysfunction, and psoriasis; a bad friendship! ***Int J Dermatol. 2018. doi: 10.1111/ijd.14178.***

Abstract

Chronic systemic diseases have a role in erectile dysfunction. Male psoriasis patients are also known to have a decreased serum testosterone levels and a higher level of estradiol as compared to individuals without psoriasis. In this study, 50 male psoriatic patients and 30 controls were studied. The erectile function and the serum total testosterone and estradiol levels were measured in all the subjects.

COMMENT

There are various pathogenic mechanisms of psoriasis. Sex hormones also have an immunological and biologic effect on the skin and thus may play a role in psoriasis pathogenesis. Loss of sexual function has a significant impact on the quality of life of patients.

In this study, the levels of sex hormones and the erectile function were studied in 50 male patients with psoriasis and 30 controls without psoriasis.

Enzyme-linked immunosorbent assay (ELISA) was used to measure the serum total testosterone and estradiol levels in all the patients. Erectile function of all patients was assessed with the help of version-5 International Index for Erectile Function.

There was a lower testosterone and higher estradiol levels in patients of psoriasis as compared to controls. This finding is corresponding with the results of other studies as well. Moreover, patients with psoriasis also had significantly more impairment of erectile function as compared to controls.

Further studies in larger number of patients are needed to confirm these findings.

Key Message

- ***Erectile dysfunction in patients with psoriasis may be due to a hormonal imbalance i.e. decreased testosterone and increased estradiol levels apart from the role of chronic systemic disease in disrupting erectile function.***

ARTICLE 63

Psoriasis and Suicidality: A Systematic Review and Meta-analysis

Singh S, Taylor C, Kornmehl H, et al. Psoriasis and suicidality: A systematic review and meta-analysis.
J Am Acad Dermatol. 2017; 77(3):425-40.e2.

Abstract

Psoriasis is a chronic inflammatory disease with psychiatric comorbidities. This study was performed to provide a systemic review and meta-analysis to determine the relationship between psoriasis and suicidality. A total of 18 studies were selected and it was found that patients with psoriasis were more likely to exhibit suicidal behaviors (combined attempted and completed suicides) with a pooled OR of 1.26. It was also found that younger patients had more likelihood for suicidal tendencies. The limitation was that there were few studies which show the conjunction of suicidality with psoriasis severity.

COMMENT

Though psoriasis is usually asymptomatic, the lesions particularly over the scalp may present with intense itching and the lesions over the palms and soles are very painful due to fissuring and hence there is significant impairment in the quality of life (QOL). It is a well known fact that any form of stress aggravates the disease process and the important is the psychological stress because of the disease process which in turn aggravates the severity of the disease. Because of the cosmetic disfigurement and the misconception of the disease as a contagious one may lead to social isolation, job displacement and family problems which finally culminate into depression.

According to studies, psoriasis patients commonly suffer from depression than the normal population. Literature reveals that prevalence of psoriasis patients resorting to suicidal tendencies is high. The term suicidality can be illustrated by the thoughts of suicide, any attempt to commit suicide or any attempt of suicide which eventually culminates. Suicidal behavior can be termed when there is an attempt to suicide or a completed act. This study aims to compile or present data regarding suidality and psoriasis.

The analysis was done by applying the Preferred Reporting Items for Systematic Reviews and Meta-analyses guidelines and by systematically searching the PubMed, EMBASE, PsycINFO, and Cochrane databases. Also, the literature published between 1946 and 2017 were analyzed.

The study found that the incidence rate of psoriasis patients who completed suicide was higher than the control population. In the studies taken for analysis, it was found that suicidality was higher in the psoriasis patients who were in their second and third decade. Also the thoughts to commit suicide and attempting to it are considerably higher in psoriasis patients who suffer from severe disease.

The possible explanation for the depression and suicidal ideation in patients of psoriasis can be explained by the fact that there is increased levels of interleukins 1, 6, 17 and tumor necrosis factor alpha in the CSF of psoriasis patients which in turn may interfere in the metabolism of serotonin leading to the depression and suicidal tendencies.

Key Messages

- *The incidence rate of psoriasis patients who completed suicide was higher than the control population*
- *The elevated levels of interleukins 1, 6, 17 and TNF-a in the CSF of psoriasis patients makes them more prone for depression and suicidal tendencies*
- *Apart from dermatological treatment adequate psychological support is required in psoriasis patients who suffer from severe disease.*

ARTICLE 64

Psoriasis and Vitiligo are Close Relatives

Sharquie KE, Salman HA, Yaseen AK. Psoriasis and vitiligo are close relatives.
Clin Cosmet Investig Dermatol. 2017;10:341-5.

Abstract

Vitiligo and psoriasis are chronic diseases which have a genetic component. This study was performed to determine the frequencies of psoriasis in vitiligo patients and vice versa and to compare them with healthy controls. A total of 1000 subjects were taken, of which 250 had vitiligo, 250 had psoriasis and 500 were chosen as healthy controls. The frequency of psoriasis among vitiligo patients was 15 and the frequency of vitiligo among psoriatic patients was 5. This study shows the close relationship between vitiligo and psoriasis.

COMMENT

Psoriasis and vitiligo can be considered as close relatives in the sense that both are medicated by T helper 1 cell mediated disorders with differences in clinical presentation. Psoriasis is a papulosquamous disorder where there is increased shedding of stratum corneum visible as scales while vitiligo is characterized by depigmented patches due to absence of melanocytes, the etiology of which is many.

The study was performed to determine the incidence of psoriasis in patients of vitiligo and the incidence of vitiligo occurring in patients of psoriasis. The study population was 1000 of which 500 were taken as controls. Other than the above-mentioned objective, the family history of development of psoriasis in vitiligo patients and vice versa was analyzed.

The study observed that the occurrence of vitiligo in psoriasis patients was seen in 2% of the patients. It was also noted that when the patients of vitiligo were inquired about the family history of psoriasis, it was found to be statistically significant. Also, the family history of vitiligo in psoriasis patients was highly significant.

Close analysis of results had shown that patients with vitiligo had a higher chance to develop psoriasis while patients with psoriasis had a lower chance to develop vitiligo as frequency of psoriasis among vitiligo patients was 6% while the frequency of vitiligo among psoriasis was 2% only.

Key Messages

The documents in favor of close link between vitiligo and psoriasis are as follows:

- *Genetic and immunological factors are present in both the diseases*
- *The two major skin diseases share a common genetic locus in the MHC*
- *Th1 cytokines play a role in the etiopathogenesis of both the diseases.*

ARTICLE 65

Psoriasis Is Associated with Risk of Obstructive Sleep Apnea Independently from Metabolic Parameters and Other Comorbidities: A Large Hospital-based Case-control Study

Papadavid E, Dalamaga M, Vlami K, et al. Psoriasis is associated with risk of obstructive sleep apnea independently from metabolic parameters and other comorbidities: A large hospital-based case-control study. ***Sleep Breath. 2017;21(4):949-58.***

Abstract

The association between obstructive sleep apnea (OSA) and psoriasis in literatures are limited. This hospital-based case-control study was performed to determine the inverse relationship, that is whether psoriasis might represent an independent predictor of OSA and its severity considering important predisposing factors. The study showed that the prevalence of psoriasis was higher in OSA patients and not associated with the severity or sleep efficacy. Therefore, psoriasis may represent an independent risk factor for OSA.

COMMENT

Psoriasis, in particular in the moderate to severe form, is a common systemic inflammatory disease with increasing prevalence, and is associated with significant morbidity and mortality. Sleep apnea is a chronic condition in which the upper respiratory airways intermittently collapse during sleep, leading to episodes of hypoxia that can trigger systemic inflammation, sympathetic nervous system activation, metabolic dysregulation, endothelial dysfunction, and increased coagulation. Sleep apnea is recognized as an important cause of cardiovascular morbidity and mortality, cognitive dysfunction, impaired work performance, and reduced quality of life.

Literature about the relation between obstructive sleep apnea (OSA) and psoriasis are very few. This study has been conducted to analyze the relationship between psoriasis and OSA, and the type of psoriasis associated with OSA.

This hospital-based study was done to evaluate the above mentioned objective with the use of clinical examination and polysomnography. It was found that OSA is prevalent considerably higher in cases of psoriasis.

The presentation of OSA in psoriatic and non-psoriatic patients is similar and moreover does not have any relation with the PASI score. However, psoriatic individuals were less compliant with CPAP treatment as compared to those without psoriasis. The reason for which has to be further studied and investigated.

The activities of the proinflammatory transcription factor in the interleukin (IL)-17 signaling pathway and nuclear factor (NF)-κB, and systemic concentrations of downstream inflammatory cytokines such as tumor necrosis factor (TNF)-α and IL-6, respectively, are significantly increased in patients with sleep apnea compared to obese controls; and in patients with psoriasis, circulating levels of TNF-α, IL-6, and IL-17 have been positively correlated with disease severity.

Key Messages

- *The presentation of OSA in psoriatic and non-psoriatic patients is similar and moreover does not have any relation with the PASI score*
- *However, psoriatic individuals were less compliant with CPAP treatment as compared to those without psoriasis.*

ARTICLE 66

Psoriasis, Fracture Risk and Bone Mineral Density: The HUNT Study, Norway

Modalsli E, Åsvold B, Romundstad P, et al. Psoriasis, fracture risk and bone mineral density: The HUNT Study, Norway. ***Br J Dermatol. 2017;176(5):1162-9.***

Abstract

This prospective population-based Norwegian study was performed to determine whether psoriasis is associated with decrease in the bone mineral density. In this study, a total of 48,194 participants in HUNT 3 trial were assessed. There was increased risk of forearm or hip fracture in 2,804 patients with psoriasis. No clear association was found between psoriasis and mean BMD T-score; overall age- and sex-adjusted differences in total hip, femoral neck and lumbar spine BMD T-scores.

COMMENT

Psoriasis is associated with other chronic inflammatory skin diseases like Crohn's disease and psoriatic arthritis. An association between psoriasis and osteoporosis has been reported and chronic inflammation has been put forward as the link between psoriasis and several comorbidities, including osteoporosis. Fractures are main clinical consequence of osteoporosis and associated with high morbidity and mortality.

The study was conducted to determine the association of psoriasis with bone mineral density and whether it is associated with increased risk for fracture of the hip or forearm.

In this study, there was no increased risk of fracture in psoriasis patients. No clear association was found between psoriasis and prevalent osteoporosis in total hip, femoral neck or lumbar spine; overall age- and sex-adjusted odds ratio was 0.77.

A major strength in this study is the population-based design which provided information less prone for bias and also the large sample size contributed to more precise estimates. The broad range of information in the HUNT study enabled to examine potential confounding factors like educational status, smoking and steroid use.

The limitation of this study is the use of self-reported psoriasis not diagnosed by a physician or a dermatologist. The majority of false-positive cases had a history of psoriasis which was not verified by a dermatologist or previous skin biopsy. Another limitation is the high number of non-participants in the bone densitometry analysis.

Key Messages

- ***No association between psoriasis and risk of fracture was found in this study***
- ***The study did not indicate reduced BMD T-score or higher prevalence of osteoporosis among patients with psoriasis***
- ***The findings suggest no need for increased awareness of osteoporosis and fracture risk among people with psoriasis in the general population.***

ARTICLE 67

Rate of Serious Infection in Patients Who Are Prescribed Systemic Biologic or Nonbiologic Agents for Psoriasis: A Large, Single Center, Retrospective, Observational Cohort Study

Carneiro C, Bloom R, Ibler E, et al. Rate of serious infection in patients who are prescribed systemic biologic or nonbiologic agents for psoriasis: A large, single center, retrospective, observational cohort study.
***Dermatol Ther*. 2017;30(5):e12529.**

Abstract

This large, single center, retrospective, observational cohort study was conducted to determine whether the systemic biologic and nonbiologic agents used to treat psoriasis may or may not contribute to serious infection (SI) risk. A total of 1,346 patients were exposed to systemic agent for psoriasis and serious infection was observed in 27 patients. The study found no statistically significant difference for risk of serious infection in patients prescribed biological/non-biological treatment for psoriasis.

COMMENT

Psoriasis is a chronic immune-mediated disorder that often requires long-term treatment, with conventional systemic therapy or biologic therapies. Biologic and conventional systemic agents used for treating psoriasis may be associated with an increased risk of serious infection; however, the degrees of risk may differ with each therapy.

Predisposition to infection in patients on biologic therapy have been studied in patients with rheumatoid arthritis and Crohn's disease. However, these inflammatory disorders by itself have higher prevalence of infection as compared to psoriasis.

The treatment of psoriasis and other disorder like Crohn's disease may be different because patient of other inflammatory disorders are usually given other chemotherapeutic agents thereby predisposing them to acquire any infection.

Among the biologicals TNF-α inhibitors are associated with higher rate of acquiring infection compared to IL-12/23 inhibitors.

Increasing age, diabetes mellitus, history of significant infection, and the use of tobacco were also significantly associated with serious infections. However, comparing biologic and nonbiologic agent exposure, no statistically significant difference for risk of SI was detectable.

In this population, the SI rate for biologic and nonbiologic systemic agents was clinically indistinguishable, thereby supporting consideration of the entire spectrum of available systemic therapeutic agents, both biologic and nonbiologic agents, for management of moderate to severe psoriasis.

Key Message

- ***Not much significant difference in the serious infection rate was observed between biological and non-biological therapies.***

ARTICLE 68

Review of Phase III Trial Data on IL-23 Inhibitors Tildrakizumab and Guselkumab for Psoriasis

Amin M, Darji K, No DJ, et al. Review of phase III trial data on IL-23 inhibitors tildrakizumab and guselkumab for psoriasis. *J Eur Acad Dermatol Venereol. 2017;31(10):1627-32.*

Abstract

Recent development of monoclonal antibodies which target IL-12 and IL-23 has enhanced the therapeutic options for psoriasis patients. The objective was to review the phase III clinical trial data for the anti-IL-23 agents to evaluate the safety and efficacy profile of each agent. By week 12, the proportion of patients reaching Psoriasis Area and Severity Index (PASI 75) was >60% among the most efficacious dose of each agent. This study shows that IL-23 agents bring rapid clinical improvement but have a relatively short-term safety profile.

COMMENT

The development of new biologic drugs that target specific mediators in the immunopathogenesis of plaque psoriasis has transformed management of the disease and has increased the range of options beyond phototherapies and traditional immunosuppressants. Evidence is accumulating to suggest that IL-23 and its resulting Th17 pathway play a more important role in psoriasis than IL-12. Tildrakizumab is a humanized immunoglobulin (Ig) G1k monoclonal anti-IL-23p19 antibody that does not bind to IL-12 or p40. Guselkumab is a human IgG1 monoclonal anti-IL-23 antibody.

This study was performed to analyze the efficacy and adverse effects associated with the administration of tildrakizumab and guselkumab. The treatment end point for each agent was considered when psoriasis area severity index of 90 was attained in 4 months which was favorably seen with guselkumab. Both the drugs had similar side effects, the commonly noted were respiratory tract infections. Although, the effects of IL-12/IL-23 inhibitors on vascular inflammation and thrombosis, especially early in the course of therapy, remain to be determined, cardiovascular risk factors should be assessed prior to the treatment.

Emerging biologic therapies that selectively inhibit either IL-23 or IL-17 significantly reduced the severity of moderate to severe plaque psoriasis during 12–16 weeks of treatment.

Key Messages

- *The anti-IL-23 agents demonstrated a rapid clinical improvement similar or superior to the improvement seen with IL-17 inhibitors with a favorable short-term safety profile*
- *The results of the phase III trials support the notion that IL-23 is a potential target in psoriasis treatment.*

ARTICLE 69

Risk for Hepatitis B and C Virus Reactivation in Patients with Psoriasis on Biologic Therapies: A Retrospective Cohort Study and Systematic Review of the Literature

Snast I, Atzmony L, Braun M, et al. Risk for hepatitis B and C virus reactivation in patients with psoriasis on biologic therapies: A retrospective cohort study and systematic review of the literature.
J Am Acad Dermatol. 2017;77(1):88-97.

Abstract

This retrospective cohort study was performed to evaluate the safety of biologic therapies in psoriasis patients seropositive for hepatitis B or C viruses. Serology revealed HCV infection in four patients, past HBV infection in 17 patients, isolated core antibody in eight patients, and chronic HBV infection in one patient. There was no reactivation of the virus or hepatitis during the follow-up. This study shows that biological therapies pose minimal risk for viral reactivation in psoriasis patients with hepatitis B or C.

COMMENT

The important inflammatory mediator which helps in the clearance of infections like tuberculosis, leprosy and acquired immunodeficiency syndrome is tumor necrosis factor alpha. So, there is obvious explanation as to why patients treated with inhibitors of tumor necrosis factor alpha have increased propensity to develop life threatening infections.

Many studies have shown that chronic hepatitis B infected patients when administered tumor necrosis factor alpha lead to the disease being reactivated with treatment and hence few authors have suggested that administering tumor necrosis factor alpha concomitant with antiviral agents can prevent the reactivation process.

This study was performed to assess whether the patients who are positive serologically for hepatitis B and C virus can safely be administered biological drugs and to evaluate whether the disease gets reactivated with therapy. The study also evaluates the need for administering any antiviral drug can prevent the disease activation.

Due to a lack of consensus in managing HBV carriers with psoriasis or psoriatic arthritis, antiviral prophylaxis is usually used in conjunction with anti-TNF-α therapy, based on the suggestions for HBV carriers receiving chemotherapeutic agents for their malignancies. The most significant predictive factor for HBV reactivation is the HBV DNA level before the start of cytotoxic or immunosuppressive therapy. Treatment with antiviral agents such as lamivudine is usually suggested in patients with a HBV DNA level of more than 10^5 copies/mL.

In patients receiving anti-TNF-α therapy, measurements of base-line HBV DNA and AST/ALT levels as well as regular follow-up assessments of these clinical parameters are recommended for the determination of antiviral prophylaxis or early detection of HBV reactivation.

Key Messages

- ***Biologic therapies pose minimal risk for viral reactivation in low-risk patients without hepatitis seropositive for HCV or HBV core antibody***
- ***Antiviral prophylaxis is necessary in patients at considerable risk of chronic HBV infection.***

ARTICLE 70

Risk of Developing Psoriasis in Patients with Schizophrenia: A Nationwide Retrospective Cohort Study

Yu S, Yu CL, Huang YC, et al. Risk of developing psoriasis in patients with schizophrenia: A nationwide retrospective cohort study.

J Eur Acad Dermatol Venereol. 2017;31(9):1497-504.

Abstract

Schizophrenia is a complex disorder which is affected by genetic and environmental factors. Psoriasis is a chronic inflammatory disorder in which Th17 cells signaling is important in the disease pathogenesis. This Th17 signaling is also observed in patients with schizophrenia. This nationwide retrospective study was performed to investigate the association of schizophrenia and psoriasis. The results of this showed that Th17 signaling and other cytokines provide a link between psoriasis and schizophrenia.

COMMENT

Psoriasis is a T-cell mediated relapsing inflammatory disorder predominantly affecting the skin but can involve the joints and nails. The disorder is mostly asymptomatic but sometimes can present with severe itching particularly the scalp psoriasis. The quality of life can be affected because of the aforesaid symptoms and moreover the appearances of skin lesions often have severe impacts on the patient's psychological and social life. Many studies have shown the positive correlation between psychiatric disorders in patients with psoriasis. The approximate prevalence of depression in psoriatic patients can be estimated up to 15%.

The exact reason between the associations of psychiatric disorders in psoriasis patients is not known. Studies have shown that the psoriasis patients are treated more with antidepressants rather than anti-psychotics. The recent literature shows that Th17 signaling pathway which plays a main role in psoriasis pathogenesis, has also role in schizophrenia.

This study was done to determine whether patients with schizophrenia have higher risk of psoriasis. The study population comprised of patients diagnosed with schizophrenia while the comparison population comprised of enrollees who had not been diagnosed with schizophrenia during the study period. Hazard ratio (HR) and 95% confidence interval (CI) were determined for the risk of psoriasis associated with schizophrenia.

It has been described in recent articles that Th17 cells and proinflammatory cytokines which play a role in psoriasis, are also involved in the pathogenesis of schizophrenia. The activation of Th17 cells occur mostly in a fresh case of schizophrenia. The reason for how psoriatic patients develop schizophrenia is that the blood-brain barrier might be disrupted in psoriasis patients by which the Th17 acts on the brain causing schizophrenia.

Key Messages

- ***Patients with schizophrenia have higher risk of psoriasis due to common genetic susceptibilities and/ or immunologic mechanisms in both diseases***
- ***Th17 signalling and proinflammatory cytokines may act as a link between these two diseases and are potential therapeutic targets for schizophrenia.***

ARTICLE 71

Risk of Malignancy with Systemic Psoriasis Treatment in the Psoriasis Longitudinal Assessment Registry

Fiorentino D, Ho V, Lebwohl MG, et al. Risk of malignancy with systemic psoriasis treatment in the psoriasis longitudinal assessment registry.
J Am Acad Dermatol. 2017;77(5):845-54.e5.

Abstract

The systemic agents used in the treatment of moderate to severe psoriasis and development of the risk of malignancies are not known. This longitudinal assessment registry was performed to determine the risk of malignancies in patients of psoriasis who are treated with systemic agents. The results were that long-term treatment with tumor necrosis factor-α (TNF-α) inhibitors are associated with increased risk of malignancies compared to other drugs.

COMMENT

Psoriasis in the United States is common during the second decade or can occur at an older age group. Literature has shown that psoriasis patients are more prone to develop malignancies like lymphoma and non-melanoma skin cancer (NMSC), compared to those without psoriasis.

The data regarding the malignancy risk associated with the most commonly used chemotherapeutic agent like methotrexate is not much whereas the malignancy risk associated with biologicals like TNF-α inhibitors has speculated to have mixed opinions.

This study was performed to determine the risk of development of malignancies in patients of psoriasis who are administered systemic treatment. The term case was used when the patient develops any first malignancy and not nonmelanoma skin cancers and the controls were matched by age, sex and place.

The drugs studied were methotrexate, ustekinumab, and TNF-α inhibitors. The exposure period was included as 1 or more doses of treatment period within one year of onset of malignancy. Multivariate conditional logistic regression was used to estimate odds ratios of malignancies associated with therapy.

It was found that treatment with methotrexate or ustekinumab used for less than 1 year was not associated with any malignancy risk and risk of malignancy was found when they were used for more than 1 year.

The results from this study can be applied to general population as the data were collected from many tertiary care centers, various institutions and communities. The limitations are that it is not a randomized controlled trial and treatment bias could not be ruled out.

Key Message

- ***Long-term (≥12 months) treatment with a TNF-a inhibitor, but not methotrexate and ustekinumab, may increase risk for malignancy in patients with psoriasis.***

ARTICLE 72

Risk of Suicidality in People with Psoriasis: A Systematic Review and Meta-analysis of Cohort Studies

Chi CC, Chen TH, Wang SH, et al. Risk of suicidality in people with psoriasis: A systematic review and meta-analysis of cohort studies.
Am J Clin Dermatol. 2017;18(5):621-7.

Abstract

The association of psoriasis with psychiatric illnesses like depression and anxiety is well known but limited literature is available regarding the relationship between psoriasis and suicidality. This systematic review and meta-analysis of cohort studies was done to assess the risk of suicidality in patients with psoriasis. This review showed that there is no increase in the risk of suicide among patients with psoriasis. The limitation of this review is that the limited data are taken for the assessment and more studies are required in the future to avail the exact figures.

COMMENT

Psoriasis can be a debilitating disease associated with various physical and psychological symptoms. Psychological comorbidities like anxiety, depression and suicidal tendencies are seen in patients with psoriasis. Usually the severity of psychological problems correlate with the severity of the disease in which patients with milder disease have anxiety and depression whereas in severe cases, patients may have suicidal tendencies.

The pathomechanisms of psoriasis and psychological problems are interlinked. Elevated cytokine levels (IL-1 and IL-6) in the central nervous system cause physiologic and biochemical changes that may contribute to the development of depression.

This review article evaluates the risk of suicide, suicide attempt, suicidal ideation, and suicidality in people with psoriasis. This systematic review and meta-analysis of cohort studies examines the risk of suicide, suicide attempt, suicidal ideation, and suicidality in people with psoriasis.

There was no increase in the risk of suicide, suicide attempt or suicidality among people with psoriasis. In the stratified analysis, no increase in suicide, suicide attempt, and suicidality among people with either severe or mild psoriasis was found.

Patients with more severe psoriasis were more likely to contemplate and attempt suicides. Greater severity of psoriasis has been associated with greater social stigmatization, substantially impaired quality of life, and higher depression rates, all of which can contribute to greater suicidal ideation and behavior.

Key Messages

- *The available limited, very low-quality evidence does not support an association between psoriasis and suicidal thought, and behavior*
- *Further studies are needed to clarify whether a subgroup of patients with psoriasis has an elevated risk of suicidality.*

ARTICLE 73

Safety of Systemic Agents for the Treatment of Pediatric Psoriasis

Bronckers IMGJ, Seyger MMB, West DP, et al. Safety of systemic agents for the treatment of pediatric psoriasis. *JAMA Dermatol. 2017;153(11):1147-57.*

Abstract

The treatment of pediatric psoriasis with systemic agents is increasing, but data regarding their use and toxicities are limited. This retrospective review was done to assess the usage and risks associated with the use of systemic agents in children with moderate to severe psoriasis. Medication related side effects were seen less often with tumor necrosis factor inhibitor drugs. Methotrexate induced side effects like gastrointestinal involvement can be avoided by administering folic acid. A registry is required to be maintained to look for any long-term risks associated with systemic agents in children.

COMMENT

Psoriasis is a common disease affecting 2–3% of adults in the United States and Europe, with as many as one-third of them had their disease begin before the age of 18. Psoriasis incidence has two peaks, one in adolescence before 20 years of age and another in adulthood. As for adult psoriasis, pediatric psoriasis has recently been associated with obesity, metabolic syndrome, increased waist circumference percentiles and metabolic laboratory abnormalities, warranting early monitoring and lifestyle modifications.

This study was performed to determine risks associated with the use of systemic agents for moderate to severe psoriasis in children. The parameters considered were age, sex, severity of psoriasis, systemic intervention and discontinuation of drug.

There were 390 children with psoriasis in this study who were on one or more systemic medications and systemic intervention was started when the disease was present for more than 3 years duration. Methotrexate was used by majority of the patients followed by acitretin.

Out of the patients who were on methotrexate, 48% had gastrointestinal side effects. Folic acid administered daily along with methotrexate reduced the incidence of gastrointestinal AEs. Obese patients who were administered methotrexate had elevation of hepatic transaminase levels.

Injection site reactions occurred in 19% of the patients who were given tumor necrosis factor inhibitors. The discontinuation of the drug due to side effects was most commonly seen with methotrexate rather than TNF-α inhibitors.

Six patients developed a serious treatment-related AE more commonly seen with methotrexate. None of the cases developed tuberculosis or malignancies.

Key Messages

- *Medication-related AEs occur less often with tumour necrosis factor inhibitors than with methotrexate*
- *Folic acid administration 6 or 7 times per week protected more against methotrexate-induced gastrointestinal AEs than did weekly administration*
- *A prospective registry is needed to track the long-term risks of systemic agents for pediatric psoriasis.*

ARTICLE 74

Severity of Psoriasis Differs between Men and Women: A Study of the Clinical Outcome Measure Psoriasis Area and Severity Index (PASI) in 5438 Swedish Register Patients

Hägg D, Sundström A, Eriksson M, et al. Severity of psoriasis differs between men and women: A study of the clinical outcome measure Psoriasis Area and Severity Index (PASI) in 5438 Swedish register patients.
Am J Clin Dermatol. 2017;18(4):583-90.

Abstract

Psoriasis is papulosquamous disorder with metabolic and cardiovascular morbidity. Previous speculations have shown that men suffer from severe psoriasis than women and they increasingly seek medical care compared to women. This cross-sectional study was performed to investigate the sex differences in the severity of psoriasis. This study shows that women have less severe psoriasis and hence they do not require systemic treatment compared to men.

COMMENT

Psoriasis prevalence in the Western population ranges from 1–5%. Comorbidities like cardiovascular, metabolic syndrome, and depression are seen with more severe cases of psoriasis. Studies have revealed that systemic treatments were given more for males compared to females.

The study was performed was to determine any sex differences in the severity of psoriasis using the Psoriasis Area Severity Index (PASI) score.

This study collected data from the national registry for systemic treatment of psoriasis in Sweden patients with moderate to severe psoriasis.

Psoriasis Area Severity Index was analyzed to determine the disease severity. It was found that women had lower PASI compared to men. Also, the PASI score in women was low in all areas of the body except for the head. There was no differences in prior treatments before enrolment could be found which may cause this difference between the sexes.

Studies have shown that men resort to treatment from dermatologists compared to women. Also, a questionnaire-based study showed that men received more systemic treatment like retinoids, methotrexate, psoralen and ultraviolet A therapy compared to women.

Key Messages

- ***The fact that women have less severe psoriasis can explain the dominance of males in the systemic treatment of psoriasis***
- ***These findings motivate a gender perspective in the management of psoriasis and in the prevention and management of its comorbidities.***

ARTICLE 75

Silencing of Homeobox A5 Gene in the Stratum Corneum of Psoriasis

Nobeyama Y, Umezawa Y, Nakagawa H. Silencing of homeobox A5 gene in the stratum corneum of psoriasis. *Exp Dermatol. 2017;26(11):1068-74.*

Abstract

The psoriatic scales can be analysed to understand the pathogenesis of psoriasis. Genes in the stratum corneum can be silenced by DNA methylation and hence methylation analysis can be performed to understand the above mechanism. This study was performed to determine genes which are silenced in the stratum corneum. Immunohistochemical staining revealed that HOXA5 protein was not expressed in the stratum corneum of fully developed psoriatic epidermis, but the protein was expressed in the stratum corneum of incompletely developed epidermis and normal epidermis.

COMMENT

Homeobox genes are a family of similar genes that direct the formation of many body structures during early embryonic development. Homeobox genes, which often appear in clusters, are present on every human chromosome.

The parakeratotic cells of psoriasis can be analysed with methylation analysis for proper understanding of pathogenesis of psoriasis.

The present study deals with the genomic elements which are muted in the lesional skin of psoriatic patients. The study was performed to evaluate the fact that certain genes in the psoriasis skin can be muted by the process of methylation.

The study was performed by subjecting the skin of psoriasis patients and normal controls to methylation analysis using polymerase chain reaction technique. It was found that the gene Homeobox A5 was muted or not expressed in the lesional skin of psoriasis patients and not in normal skin. More studies on Homeobox A5 silencing in the pathology of psoriasis are required.

Key Messages

- *HOXA5 can be silenced in the stratum corneum of psoriasis*
- *The silenced gene was identified by non-invasive methylation analysis of psoriatic scales.*

ARTICLE 76

Skin-infiltrating, Interleukin-22-producing T cells Differentiate Pediatric Psoriasis from Adult Psoriasis

Cordoro KM, Hitraya-Low M, Taravati K, et al. Skin-infiltrating, interleukin-22–producing T cells differentiate pediatric psoriasis from adult psoriasis.
J Am Acad Dermatol. 2017;77(3):417-24.

Abstract

The role of Th-17 cells infiltrating the psoriatic plaques in adults is well known, but the role in pediatric psoriasis is not known. This study was performed to analyze the inflammatory cell profiles of psoriatic plaques in pediatric patients and compare to the adult psoriasis patients. This study shows that IL-22 might be relevant in the pathogenesis of pediatric psoriasis and represents a potential treatment target unique to pediatric psoriasis.

COMMENT

Psoriasis has a worldwide prevalence of 1–3%. Psoriasis is a frequent condition in children, but only limited epidemiologic data are available. Various published large series have reported that of all psoriasis patients, 20–35% have onset of their disease before the age of 20 years. It accounts for 4% of all dermatoses seen in children.

In adult patients with psoriasis the role of imbalance between regulatory and effector T-cells, particularly Th17 producing T-cells has been proposed. However, the immunopathology in childhood psoriasis is not known.

This study was performed to determine the inflammatory cells infiltrating the lesions of pediatric psoriasis patients and compare with the infiltrates from the lesions in adult patients with psoriasis.

In this study, in order to determine the nature of the infiltrating inflammatory subsets and the cytokines present, flow cytometry was performed using the skin samples and analyzed.

The inflammatory infiltrate in pediatric psoriasis patients comprised more of IL-22 compared to infiltrates from adult lesions which had more of IL-17. Also, lesional skin in pediatric patients with psoriasis did not have increased regulatory T-cells when compared with adults.

Key Messages

- *Differences in IL-17 and IL-22 expression were observed in the paediatric psoriasis patients compared with pediatric healthy controls and adult psoriasis patients*
- *IL-22 might be relevant in the pathogenesis of pediatric psoriasis and represents a potential treatment target unique to pediatric psoriasis.*

ARTICLE 77

Spotlight on Ixekizumab for the Treatment of Moderate-to-Severe Plaque Psoriasis: Design, Development, and Use in Therapy

Giunta A, Ventura A, Chimenti MS, et al. Spotlight on ixekizumab for the treatment of moderate-to-severe plaque psoriasis: Design, development, and use in therapy.
Drug Des Devel Ther. 2017;11:1643-51.

Abstract

In the recent years, there have been developments in the understanding of new immunopathogenesis like IL-17 as the important cytokine which can be targeted for the treatment of adults with moderate-to-severe psoriasis. Ixekizumab is the humanized monoclonal antibody which targets IL-17A used in the treatment of moderate-to-severe psoriasis. This study shows that ixekizumab brought clinical improvement and a favorable safety profile in phase III trials. Ixekizumab has characteristics of consistent efficacy and rapid onset of response which is not influenced by previous exposure to biologics and has shown good results in areas that are difficult to treat and in severe clinical variants of psoriasis.

COMMENT

Psoriasis is a chronic relapsing T cell mediated inflammatory disease with systemic associations which requires a multidisciplinary approach and an appropriated treatment taking into account different comorbidities. The recent research activities have shown the main role of IL-17 in the pathogenesis of psoriasis.

IL-17A is the main cytokine which orchestrates the events that lead to inflammation, neutrophil recruitment and interacting with other cytokines, chemokines, acute-phase proteins, antimicrobial peptides, mucins, and matrix metalloproteinases.

Ixekizumab is an anti-IL-17A biological drug which is indicated for the treatment of moderate-to-severe plaque-type psoriasis. Ixekizumab binds to human IL-17A thereby neutralizing the proinflammatory effect of IL-17A/F heterodimers. This drug is administered subcutaneously; initially 160 mg is given first ensued by 80 mg in weeks 2, 4, 6, 8, 10, and 12. After that, a maintenance dose of 80 mg is administered every 4 weeks. The mean elimination half-life of this drug is 10 days.

In this clinical trial, it was shown that a large group of study population has shown good results after drug therapy. Ixekizumab was found to have brought clinical improvement and acceptable safety profile in phase III trials. Ixekizumab is an efficacious drug with quick treatment response; the latter is not influenced by previous exposure to biologics.

The efficacy of ixekizumab is highlighted in this article as the drug is effective in moderate-to-severe psoriasis and the response does not vary with new patients or patients who have failed to other biologicals.

Key Messages

- *Ixekizumab is an effective drug with a good safety profile and multiple target profile.*
- *It could be useful in patients with severe forms of psoriasis either as a first-line therapy or second-line when not responding to other agents.*

ARTICLE 78

Systematic Review and Meta-analysis of the Association between Psoriasis and Metabolic Syndrome

Rodríguez-Zúñiga MJM, García-Perdomo HA. Systematic review and meta-analysis of the association between psoriasis and metabolic syndrome.
J Am Acad Dermatol. 2017;77(4):657-66.

Abstract

The association between psoriasis and metabolic syndrome (MS) is well known but no meta-analysis has been restricted to studies that adjusted for confounders. This systematic review and meta-analysis was done to find out the association between psoriasis and MS. There were a total of 14 papers selected which included 25,042 patients with psoriasis. It was found that MS was present in 31.4% of patients with psoriasis. Middle Eastern studies (Israel, Turkey, and Lebanon) reported a greater risk for MS than European studies (Germany, Italy, the United Kingdom, Norway, and Denmark). The limitation of the study was inconsistency between publications.

COMMENT

Psoriasis is a common Th1 and Th17-mediated chronic inflammatory disease that has been associated with metabolic syndrome, a constellation of cardiovascular risk factors including obesity, hypertension, dyslipidemia, and insulin resistance, has been implicated. Overlapping inflammatory pathways and genetic susceptibility may be potential biologic links underlying this association.

Though there are many studies conducted to assess the relation between psoriasis and metabolic syndrome (MS), no meta-analysis has been conducted to assess the confounders. Therefore, so this meta-analysis has been conducted to determine the association between psoriasis and MS.

A systematic review and meta-analysis of observational studies on psoriasis and MS in adults was performed from MEDLINE, Scopus, SciELO, Google Scholar, Science Direct, and LILACS from inception to January 2016. Random effects model meta-analysis for those studies was performed, reporting adjusted odds ratios (ORs) with 95% confidence intervals (CIs). The subgroup analysis was related to geographic location, diagnosis criteria and risk of bias.

There were a total of 14 papers selected which included 25,042 patients with psoriasis. It was found that MS was present in 31.4% of patients with psoriasis. Middle Eastern studies (Israel, Turkey, and Lebanon) reported a greater risk for MS than European studies (Germany, Italy, the United Kingdom, Norway, and Denmark).

Patients with psoriasis should be routinely screened for metabolic syndrome and treated accordingly to manage cardiometabolic risk, while clinicians should monitor potential effects on treatment efficacy and safety in patients with comorbid psoriasis and MS.

The limitation of this study is the inconsistency between publications.

Key Message

- ***Screening for metabolic syndrome should be considered by the treating dermatologist in patients of psoriasis with metabolic risk factors.***

ARTICLE 79

Th17 Inhibitors in Active Psoriatic Arthritis: A Systematic Review and Meta-analysis of Randomized Controlled Clinical Trials

Naik GS, Ming WK, Magodoro IM, et al. Th17 Inhibitors in active psoriatic arthritis: A systematic review and meta-analysis of randomized controlled clinical trials.
Dermatology. 2017;233:366-77.

Abstract

There are many biologicals available which target the IL-17 pathways which plays a main role in the pathogenesis of psoriasis. These IL-17 inhibitors could replace the tumor necrosis factor-α (TNF-α) inhibitors in the treatment of psoriasis in the future. This systematic review and meta-analysis was performed to determine the treatment effectiveness of IL-17 inhibitors compared to placebo or controls on American College of Rheumatology (ACR) 20 response at week 12 (primary objective), risk of infections, discontinuation of treatment due to adverse events, and serious adverse events during the placebo-controlled period (12-24 weeks) in adults with active PsA in published randomized controlled trials. The results showed that biologicals which target Th17 axis can produce a significant improvement in joint disease activity in psoriasis.

COMMENT

Interleukin-17A (IL-17A) has been shown to drive the development of skin lesions in psoriasis and enthesitis in psoriatic arthritis (PsA) while IL-23 induces differentiation of naive T-cells to Th17 producing more IL-17A. Since, the usage of tumor necrosis factor-α (TNF-α) inhibitors increase the risk of tuberculosis and other infections and also the effect is short-lasting, have led to the exploration of alternative strategies including Th17 pathway inhibitors to treat psoriasis and PsA.

A systematic review and meta-analysis of randomized controlled clinical trials (excluding phase 1 studies) was performed to determine the overall treatment effect of Th17 pathway inhibitors compared to placebo or active control on American College of Rheumatology (ACR) 20 response at week 12 (primary objective), risk of infections, discontinuation of treatment due to adverse events, and serious adverse events during the placebo-controlled period (12–24 weeks) in adults with active PsA in published randomized controlled trials.

Seven randomized controlled trials were included which randomized 1,718 patients to Th17 inhibitors and 840 to placebo. Patients treated with Th17 inhibitors had an RR of 2.04 for achieving an ACR 20 response at week 12 compared to placebo-treated patients. There was no evidence of publication bias. No incident cases of tuberculosis were reported.

The estimates for adverse events of interest, namely infections and serious adverse events, did not differ significantly between the active and the placebo groups. The data, however, do not point at a very high rate of side effects for infections and serious adverse effects from the active treatments. The pooled estimates for Candida infections were however higher compared to placebo but the confidence intervals were wide and included the null value.

Key Message

- *Biologics targeting IL-17 produce a significant improvement in joint disease activity with acceptable safety and tolerability for a short- term treatment.*

ARTICLE 80

The Acitretin and Methotrexate Combination Therapy for Psoriasis Vulgaris Achieves Higher Effectiveness and Less Liver Fibrosis

An J, Zhang D, Wu J, et al. The acitretin and methotrexate combination therapy for psoriasis vulgaris achieves higher effectiveness and less liver fibrosis.
Pharmacol Res. 2017;121:158-68.

Abstract

The systemic treatment of psoriasis involves the most commonly used agents like methotrexate and acitretin. The agents are commonly used alone, the combination of these agents are not commonly used for the warning regarding the hepatotoxicity of the drug interactions. This study was designed to investigate the effectiveness of such combination therapy for psoriasis vulgaris, and the potential benefit as well as side effect during the treatment. The results showed that the combination therapy was effective in decreasing the skin lesions and there was no significant alteration in the liver functions of the patients. Interestingly, such combination treatment induced lower expression of profibrotic factors in hepatic stellate cells.

COMMENT

Acitretin and methotrexate are both used widely in psoriasis. Both the drugs are however not given concurrently as their combination has been reported to have potential hepatotoxicity due to drug interactions. Acitretin is the drug of choice in pustular psoriasis and can be safely given in immunocompromised patients, where methotrexate and other immunosuppressants have to be used with caution.

Methotrexate is useful in both psoriasis and psoriatic arthritis, whereas acitretin has less benefit in psoriatic arthritis. There are not many studies regarding the safety and efficacy of combining acitretin and methotrexate in psoriasis. This study was conducted to evaluate the combination therapy of acitretin and methotrexate in the management of psoriasis vulgaris.

In this study, patients with psoriasis vulgaris were treated with acitretin, methotrexate or their combination or as control. Human keratinocytes and hepatic stellate cells were used for *in vitro* analysis.

The results revealed that combination therapy exhibited higher effectiveness in clearance of skin lesion as well as in helping to attain remission with no changes in the liver function. Also, it was found out that there was no increase in pro-fibrotic cytokines in the combination therapy group.

Key Message

- ***Acitretin-methotrexate combination therapy for psoriasis vulgaris can achieve higher effectiveness and results in less liver fibrosis.***

ARTICLE 81

The Efficacy of Biologic Therapy for the Management of Palmoplantar Psoriasis and Palmoplantar Pustulosis: A Systematic Review

Sanchez IM, Sorenson E, Levin E, et al. The efficacy of biologic therapy for the management of palmoplantar psoriasis and palmoplantar pustulosis: A systematic review.
Dermatol Ther (Heidelb). 2017;7:425-46.

Abstract

The usage of biological agents like Tumor necrosis factor (TNF) inhibitors like infliximab, adalimumab, IL-17A inhibitors like ixekizumab and secukinumab and IL-12/IL-23 inhibitors like guselkumab and ustekinumab in the treatment of chronic plaque psoriasis are well known, but little data is available regarding its safety and efficacy in pustular psoriasis. This systematic review was conducted to identify studies or case reports which both used biologic therapy for the treatment of hyperkeratotic palmoplantar psoriasis (PP), pustular PP, and palmoplantar pustulosis (PPP) and reported treatment outcomes. The results showed that adalimumab, guselkumab, ixekizumab, secukinumab, and ustekinumab all showed >80% efficacy for the treatment of hyperkeratotic PP, while infliximab and ustekinumab showed moderate efficacy for the treatment of pustular PP, and infliximab was the most efficacious treatment for PPP.

COMMENT

Palmoplantar psoriasis (PP) is a chronic, debilitating disease of the palms and/or soles that affects 11–39% of psoriasis patients. Pustular PP is a variant that includes macroscopic sterile pustules and erythema with intermixed yellow-brown macules localized to the palms and/or soles. The above mentioned diseases can cause marked physical discomfort and functional disability.

The Tumor necrosis factor-α (TNF-α) inhibitors drugs include infliximab, adalimumab and etanercept, IL-17A inhibitors are ixekizumab and secukinumab, and the IL-23 or IL-12/IL-23 inhibitors guselkumab and ustekinumab have been well studied for the treatment of moderate-to-severe plaque psoriasis. Data regarding the efficacy and safety of these agents for the treatment of PP (hyperkeratotic and pustular forms) and palmoplantar pustulosis (PPP) is very less.

This review was performed to study the efficacy and safety of the above mentioned biologicals in the treatment of palmoplantar psoriasis and pustular psoriasis of the palms and soles. In this review, studies which used biologic therapy for the treatment of hyperkeratotic PP, pustular PP and PPP were chosen.

The randomized controlled trials on the treatment of hyperkeratotic PP agents like adalimumab, guselkumab, infliximab, ixekizumab, and secukinumab showed greater improvement compared to placebo.

In the management of pustular PP, ustekinumab 45 mg did not show marked results though few studies have shown that that four of five patients on ustekinumab 90 mg had clinical clearance at 16 weeks. Similarly, in the treatment of PPP, etanercept and ustekinumab 45 mg did not bring about the desired results.

The analysis of studies on PPP showed that infliximab had the greatest efficacy at 100% in the clinical improvement of patients from case reports which was ensued by ustekinumab at 59% clinical improvement. Adverse effects were noted in patients treated with infliximab and secukinumab.

Key Messages

- ***Adalimumab, guselkumab, ixekizumab, secukinumab, and ustekinumab showed > 80% efficacy for the treatment of hyperkeratotic PP***
- ***Infliximab and ustekinumab showed moderate efficacy for the treatment of pustular PP***
- ***Infliximab was the most efficacious treatment for PPP.***

ARTICLE 82

The Metabolic Analysis of Psoriasis Identifies the Associated Metabolites while Providing Computational Models for the Monitoring of the Disease

Ottas A, Fishman D, Okas TL, et al. The metabolic analysis of psoriasis identifies the associated metabolites while providing computational models for the monitoring of the disease.
Arch Dermatol Res. 2017;309:519-28.

Abstract

Metabolomics is newly developing field which investigates the role of substances like amino acids, lipids and carbohydrates and their derivatives in the pathology of a disease. This study was conducted to discover the role of small molecules in the contribution to the metabolomic profile of psoriasis which in turn can be used in the future as markers to classify the severity of disease.

COMMENT

Metabolomics is newly developing field which investigates the role of substances like amino acids, lipids and carbohydrates and their derivatives in the pathology of a disease.

It has been discovered that alterations in free-circulating amino acids for example, arginine, proline, alanine, glutamate and others are increased when the plasma sample of a psoriasis patient is analyzed. The elevated levels of the above mentioned amino acids revert back to normal after treatment with Tumor necrosis factor-α (TNF-α) inhibitors.

This study was conducted to discover the role of small molecules in the contribution to the metabolomic profile of psoriasis which in turn can be used in the future as markers to classify the severity of disease.

To identify the small molecules, fasting blood samples of the patients were collected and serum was separated and then it was frozen and mass spectrographic analysis was performed to quantitate the metabolites.

Significant changes were found in the levels of acylcarnitines, phosphatidylcholines, amino acids, urea and 1,11-undecanedicarboxylic acid.

This study found that the levels of non-essential amino acids with the exception of phenylalanine were found at different concentrations. Ornithine, arginase were elevated in psoriatic skin whereas carnitines and acylcarnitines were decreased in the lesional psoriatic skin.

The molecular changes were found in the filagrin whose mRNA is expressed at a lower levels in the lesional skin. Also the ratio of citrulline to ornithine and putrescine to ornithine were altered.

The increased levels of methionine-sulfoxide can be a marker for increased oxidative stress in psoriasis. Similarly, the raised levels of phytanic acid can serve as an indicator of continued inflammation and thereby contributing to the oxidative stress in psoriaisis. The higher mitotic index of the psoriatic skin can be due to decreased concentration of phosphatidyl cholines.

Key Messages

- ***Patients with psoriasis have an impaired amino acid and lipid metabolism, and a disbalance in the components of the bilipid cellular membrane***
- ***These findings will help to understand the pathogenesis of the disease which could lead to the better treatment of patients.***

ARTICLE 83

The Relationship between Duration of Psoriasis, Vascular Inflammation and Cardiovascular Events

Egeberg A, Skov L, Joshi AA, et al. The relationship between duration of psoriasis, vascular inflammation, and cardiovascular events.
J Am Acad Dermatol. 2017;77(4):650-6.

Abstract

The association between psoriasis and cardiovascular disease is known but data regarding the duration of psoriasis affects the risk of vascular inflammation and major adverse cardiovascular events is not known. This study was performed to understand the effects of psoriasis duration on vascular disease and cardiovascular events by imaging using fludeoxyglucose F 18 positron emission tomography/computed tomography. The results showed that there is detrimental effect on the duration of psoriasis and major adverse cardiovascular event.

COMMENT

Patients with psoriasis have an increased incidence and prevalence of cardiovascular (CV) risk factors and CV disease (CVD). Vascular inflammation by fludeoxyglucose F 18 (18-FDG) positron emission tomography/computed tomography (18-FDG PET/CT), which is prognostic for future CV events, is increased in patients with psoriasis.

This study utilized two resources to understand the effect of psoriasis duration on vascular disease and CV events: (1) a human imaging study and (2) a population-based study of CVD events. First, patients with psoriasis underwent 18-FDG PET/CT. Second, major adverse cardiovascular event (MACE) risk was examined by using nationwide registries versus the general population.

In the human imaging study, patients were young, of low CV risk by traditional risk scores, and had a high prevalence of cardiometabolic diseases. Vascular inflammation by 18-FDG PET/CT was significantly associated with disease duration. In the population-based study, psoriasis duration had strong relationship with MACE risk.

Studies have shown that patients with psoriasis have an increased risk to develop CVD, the reason behind this is the role of systemic inflammation. This systemic inflammation causes the cycle of events like impaired insulin sensitivity, endothelial dysfunction and vascular inflammation. The above events can also occur consequent to immune activation in those with longer duration of disease.

Key Messages

- *Detrimental effects of psoriasis duration on vascular inflammation and MACE was found*
- *This suggests that cumulative duration of exposure to low-grade chronic inflammation may accelerate vascular disease development and MACEs.*
- *Providers should consider inquiring about duration of disease to counsel for heightened CVD risk in psoriasis.*

ARTICLE 84

The Relevance of Serum Vitamin D in Psoriasis: A Review

Hambly R, Kirby B. The relevance of serum vitamin D in psoriasis: A review.
Arch Dermatol Res. 2017;309:499-517.

Abstract

The role of vitamin D in skeletal diseases is well known. It has been found that low serum levels of vitamin D are found in general population and that supplementing vitamin D may help in reducing the mortality in elderly women and also cancer mortality. This study was conducted to review the literature to identify the relevance of serum 25(OH)D levels in psoriasis. Most of the studies which has been chosen for this review showed low levels of vitamin D in psoriasis. Multiple studies report an improvement in psoriasis with vitamin D supplementation. Low serum 25(OH)D levels may be associated with comorbidities in psoriasis patients, including metabolic syndrome and cardiovascular risk. Though there are reports that low levels of vitamin D results in many disorders, the evidence for causality is unknown.

COMMENT

Vitamin D (25-hydroxyvitamin D) is a hormone whose synthesis is stimulated by cutaneous exposure to ultraviolet B radiation. It acts on calcium homeostasis, on bone metabolism and has immune regulating functions that have been recently recognized. Some studies have demonstrated a relationship between vitamin D deficiency and psoriasis.

Studies have shown decreased serum levels of 25-hydroxyvitamin D (25[OH]D) in diseases not involving the bones. Research articles have shown the benefit of vitamin D supplementation in decreasing mortality in elderly women.

This study reviews to determine the relevance of serum 25[OH]D levels in psoriasis. The studies from which the data were collected, showed decreased vitamin D levels in psoriasis patients which reverted back to normal with phototherapy treatment. However, the increase in vitamin D levels with phototherapy does not indicate reduction in disease severity.

The adequate dosage of vitamin D to be supplemented in psoriasis patients differs between studies and exact dosing schedule is not available.

Key Messages

- *Low serum 25[OH]D levels may be associated with comorbidities in psoriasis patients, including metabolic syndrome and cardiovascular risk*
- *Supplementation in patients with low 25[OH]D is of benefit to those at risk of impaired bone health.*

ARTICLE 85

The Risk of Malignancy among Biologic-naïve Pediatric Psoriasis Patients: A Retrospective Cohort Study in a US Claims Database

Gu Y, Nordstrom BL. The risk of malignancy among biologic-naïve pediatric psoriasis patients: A retrospective cohort study in a US claims database.
J Am Acad Dermatol. 2017;77(2):293-301.

Abstract

The literature regarding the risk of malignancies in adult psoriasis is available but the data regarding the malignancy in pediatric psoriasis patients are not available. This retrospective cohort study was performed to compare the malignancy risk in biologic-naïve pediatric psoriasis patients with a matched pediatric population without psoriasis. Among 9,045 pediatric psoriasis patients and 77,206 comparators, 18 probable or highly probable cancers were identified. The results showed that there was not significant increase in cancer risk in pediatric patients compared with those patients without psoriasis but there was significant increase in lymphoma risk when compared to general population.

COMMENT

Psoriasis is a multifactorial papulosquamous disorder though commonly seen in adults is increasingly seen in the pediatric population in the recent years. Approximately 1% of the pediatric population in European countries has psoriasis.

The management of pediatric psoriasis is different from adult psoriasis wherein due consideration has to be given in controlling the severity of the disease with safer drugs. Also, the treatment has to be instituted early to prevent the comorbidities which are associated with psoriasis.

This study was conducted to identify any risk of malignancies developing in pediatric patients in whom the treatment with biological agents were given for the first time compared with normal pediatric population as controls.

There were about 18 cases of malignancies identified in this study from the 9,045 pediatric psoriasis patients. Pediatric psoriasis patients showed increased lymphoma rate when compared with the American Surveilance, Epidemiology and End Results (SEER) group and not with comparative population.

Key Messages

- ***Patients with pediatric psoriasis showed no significant increase in overall cancer risk compared with those without psoriasis***
- ***A potential increased risk for lymphoma was observed when compared with the general population.***

ARTICLE 86

Risk of Venous Thromboembolism in Patients with Psoriatic Arthritis, Psoriasis and Rheumatoid Arthritis: A General Population-based Cohort Study

Ogdie A, Kay McGill N, Shin DB, et al. Risk of venous thromboembolism in patients with psoriatic arthritis, psoriasis and rheumatoid arthritis: A general population-based cohort study.
Eur Heart J. 2017. doi: 10.1093/eurheartj/ehx145

Abstract

Venous thromboembolism (VTE) is a common and fatal condition and this study was performed to determine the risk of VTE among patients with psoriatic arthritis, psoriasis and rheumatoid arthritis (RA). This is a cohort study performed in the UK with data from 1994 to 2014 among the patients with the aforesaid conditions. The results of this study were that patients with RA and patients with mild psoriasis had a significantly elevated risk of VTE after adjusting for traditional risk factors.

Although, the risk factor for VTE is systemic inflammation which is present in all the three conditions, the risk of developing VTE differs in the three conditions.

COMMENT

Venous thromboembolism (VTE) is a relatively common and potentially fatal condition with an incidence of three cases per 1,000 patient years. One such potential risk factor for VTE is systemic inflammation. Previous studies have suggested an increased risk of VTE among patients with elevated serum C-reactive protein (CRP), interleukin-6 (IL-6), IL-8, monocyte chemotactic protein (MCP)-1 and tumor necrosis factor (TNF).

Psoriasis, psoriatic arthritis (PsA) and rheumatoid arthritis (RA) are chronic inflammatory diseases. These disorders result in activation of both the Th1 and Th17 inflammatory pathways resulting in increased IL-6 and TNF and patients often have an elevated CRP.

This study was performed to evaluate the risk of VTE defined as the combined endpoint of deep venous thrombosis (DVT) and pulmonary embolism (PE) among patients with PsA, psoriasis and RA compared with population controls.

This was a cohort study conducted in a primary care medical record database in the UK with data from 1994 to 2014 among patients with PsA, RA, or psoriasis.

An interaction with disease modifying anti-rheumatic drugs (DMARD) was hypothesized *a priori* and was significant. Patients with RA (with and without a DMARD prescription) and patients with mild psoriasis had significantly elevated risks of VTE after adjusting for traditional risk factors.

Severe psoriasis and PsA prescribed a DMARD had an elevated but not statistically significant risk for VTE. Findings were similar for DVT. The age-and-sex-adjusted risk of PE was elevated in RA, severe psoriasis and PsA patients prescribed a DMARD.

Strengths of this study include the use of a large population-based medical record database, broadly representative of the UK general population, the relatively large number of patients with PsA, psoriasis and RA, validation of the codes for the exposures and outcomes, and an unexposed cohort sampled from the general population.

Limitations of the study include the risk of exposure misclassification. Lack of direct measures of disease activity limited the assessment of active inflammation and the relationship with VTE. Similarly, not all laboratory results are available and approximately 20% of the cohort had CRP and/or sedimentation rate results.

Key Messages

- ***This study found an increased age and sex adjusted risk for VTE in patients with RA, psoriasis and PsA***
- ***This risk remained significantly elevated after adjustment for established VTE risk factors in RA and mild psoriasis***
- ***Clinicians should be aware of the increased risk of VTE and consider the diagnosis of PE or DVT in patients presenting with acute shortness of breath or acute lower extremity swelling.***

ARTICLE 87

A 2-Year Observational Study on Treatment Targets in Psoriatic Arthritis Patients Treated with TNF Inhibitors

Chimenti MS, Triggianese P, Conigliaro P, et al. A 2-year observational study on treatment targets in psoriatic arthritis patients treated with TNF inhibitors.
Clin Rheumatol. 2017;36(10):2253-60.

Abstract

Tumor necrosis factor inhibitors (TNFi) are used in the treatment of psoriasis and psoriatic arthritis. In this study the clinical remission and minimal disease activity of patients on TNFi treatment were studied with a 2-year follow-up.

A total of 221 psoriatic arthritis patients were studied. The comorbidities were also noted down. The patients were studied at baseline and at 22, 54 and 102 weeks of treatment. The parameters assessed were CPDAI, DAS28, DAPSA, HAQ-SpA and MDA.

COMMENT

This article is an observational study to evaluate the response to treatment of psoriatic arthritis (PsA) patients with Tumor necrosis factor inhibitors (TNFi) with a follow-up of 2 years. The sample size was 221.

The comorbidities and the therapies given concomitantly were also evaluated.

The minimal disease activity and the positive predictive factors for remission were evaluated. The parameters used to assess disease activity and disability were Disease activity score in 28 joints (DAS28),

Composite Psoriatic Disease Activity Index (CPDAI), Disease activity in psoriatic arthritis (DAPSA), Health assessment questionnaire-spondyloarthropathy (HAQ-SpA) and minimal disease activity (MDA). Evaluations were done at baseline and after 22, 54 and 102 weeks of treatment.

The most common risk factors were metabolic syndrome (MetS) and cardiovascular diseases. More than half the patients achieved clinical remission which further reduced the usage of steroids and disease modifying anti-rheumatoid drugs (DMARDs) at follow-up. All the evaluation parameters of treatment mentioned above showed a significant improvement at follow-up. Metabolic syndrome and female gender showed less probability to achieve remission of PsA on follow-up.

A study on a larger subset of patients is required to confirm the results of this study. The outcome on skin findings using Psoriasis Area Severity Index (PASI) could also have been done. Psoriatic arthritis screening and evaluation (PASE) and CASPAR (ClASsification criteria for Psoriatic Arthritis) could also have been done. The methods by which the diagnosis of PsA was made is not mentioned. The TNFi used in the study and the dosage needs to be mentioned.

Key Messages

- *The parameters used to assess disease activity and disability of PsA namely DAS28, CPDAI, DAPSA, HAQ-SpA and MDA showed significant improvement on treatment with tumour necrosis factor inhibitors even at 2-year follow-up*
- *Remission of PsA was noted in more than half the patients which in turn reduced the dosage of DMARDs and steroids at follow-up*
- *Female gender and metabolic syndrome showed less probability to attain PsA remission.*

ARTICLE 88

Anthralin Modulates the Expression Pattern of Cytokeratins and Antimicrobial Peptides by Psoriatic Keratinocytes

Holstein J, Fehrenbacjer B, Brück J, et al. Anthralin modulates the expression pattern of cytokeratins and antimicrobial peptides by psoriatic keratinocytes.
J Dermatol Sci. 2017;87(3):236-45.

Abstract

Psoriasis is a chronic inflammatory skin disorder with abnormal keratinocyte proliferation occurring as a result of immune cell activation. Th17 cytokines leads to epidermal thickening, altered keratinocyte differentiation and production of antimicrobial peptides. Anti-cytokine antibodies and anthralin have been used for the treatment of psoriasis. The objective of this study was to find out the effects of anthralin of keratinocyte proliferation, differentiation and the production of psoriasis associated factors.

COMMENT

This article is a study on the effects of anthralin on the differentiation and proliferation of keratinocytes and production of psoriasis associated factors.

The effects on anthralin on cytokeratin expression, antimicrobial peptide expression and cell proliferation were studies on monolayer cultures and multilayer cultures (3D models) of psoriatic tissue.

Stimulation with psoriasis promoting cytokines such as Interleukin (IL)17A and IL-22 were done and the findings on treatment with anthralin with and without stimulation were noted. The *in vitro* findings were compared to the *in vivo* findings i.e. lesional skin of psoriatic patients pre and post-treatment with anthralin.

Anthralin induced apoptosis in *in vitro* monolayer cultures but not in multilayer cultures treated/stimulated with IL-17A and IL-22. Keratinocyte proliferation assessed by Ki-67 staining was decreased subsequent to anthralin therapy in lesional skin *in vivo*.

Cytokeratin 16 (CK-16) expression was normalized by anthralin in lesional skin, but not in multilayer models. CK-16 is generally upregulated in benign keratinocyte hyperplasia including psoriasis.

Anthralin had a direct inhibitory action on Defensin Beta 4 gene (DEFB4) expression both *in vitro* and *in vivo*. Defensin Beta 4 gene encodes a protein known as Beta-defensin 2 (BD-2) which is otherwise known as skin-antimicrobial peptide (SAP1). The skin beta-defensins have antimicrobial and pro-inflammatory nature due to cytokine like properties. These cytokine-like properties lead it to being a precipitating factor of psoriasis after any skin injury, infection or environmental trigger. The other cytokines and antimicrobial peptides showed different response to anthralin *in vivo* and *in vitro*.

This study provides useful information on the mechanism of action of anthralin in psoriasis. Except for DEFB4, all the actions were different *in vitro* and *in vivo*. However, most of the *in vivo* response of psoriasis to anthralin was positive.

Key Messages

- *An inhibitory action on DEFB4 is observed both in vivo and in vitro on treatment with anthralin*
- *Keratinocyte differentiation and cytokine expression showed varying results in vivo and in vitro on anthralin treatment and a good response was predominantly seen in vivo.*

ARTICLE 89

Association of Psoriasis and Psoriatic Arthritis with Osteoporosis and Pathological Fractures

Kathuria P, Gordon KB, Silverberg JI. Association of psoriasis and psoriatic arthritis with osteoporosis and pathological fractures.
J Am Acad Dermatol. 2017;76(6):1045-53.

Abstract

The studies done previously evaluating the relationship between psoriasis, osteoporosis and pathological fractures gave varying results. This study was done with an objective of determining the association of psoriasis with fractures and osteoporosis. A pooled analysis was done across 7 years and 198,102,435 patients were studied from the National Emergency Department Sample. Psoriatic arthritis and psoriasis were associated with osteoporosis, osteopenia, pathologic fractures and ankylosing spondylitis.

COMMENT

This article is an analysis to find out the relationship between psoriasis, psoriatic arthritis (PsA) with osteoporosis and pathological fractures. Previous studies analyzing the same showed varying results.

This was a cross-sectional study and samples were taken from the National Emergency Department Sample and included 20% of emergency care visits. A total of 198,102,435 individuals were taken for the study in which 183,725 had psoriasis and 28,765 had psoriatic arthritis. The remaining were non-psoriatics.

When an analysis was done, psoriatic patients had significantly increased odds of having osteomalacia, osteopenia, pathological fractures and ankylosing spondylitis. Similar results were seen in patients with PsA.

In this study, a lot of the study subject's data were taken from emergency care visits. The majority of emergency care visits involve trauma which could be a reason for the fractures. A sample taken from an outpatient department would be more useful to come to this result.

Moreover, the mechanism by which osteopenia and osteomalacia were detected has not been mentioned.

Key Message

- ***There is increased risk of osteopenia, osteoporosis, ankylosing spondylitis, and pathologic fractures in psoriasis and psoriatic arthritis patients.***

ARTICLE 90

Associations between Body Mass Index and Severity of Psoriasis

Sobhan M, Farshchian M. Associations between body mass index and severity of psoriasis.
Clin Cosmet Investig Dermatol. 2017;10:493-498.

Abstract

Obesity and overweight have been associated with chronic skin conditions such as psoriasis. The objective of this study was to study the relationship between obesity and severity of psoriasis. A total of 42 patients were studied. Psoriasis was split into mild, moderate and severe based on the PASI score. Waist size, body mass index, gender, age, smoking and drinking habits were also recorded. There was no significant effect of age, gender, waist circumference and body mass index on the severity of psoriasis.

COMMENT

This article is a study on the relationship between obesity and psoriasis. Psoriasis is known to be associated with metabolic syndrome. Obesity has known to be a risk factor in precipitating and aggravating psoriasis.

This was a cross-sectional study in which 42 patients were studied and their data were analyzed. Psoriasis Area Severity Index (PASI) was used to divide the patients into mild (0–7), moderate (7–12) and severe (>12) disease. The other parameters studied were waist size, body mass index (BMI), gender, age and habits such as drinking and smoking.

There was no significant relation between the severity of the disease and the BMI or waist circumference. Moreover, there was no significant effect on habits such as smoking and drinking on the severity of the disease.

A study with a larger sample size would be useful in confirmation of the above findings since in most of the studies on obesity and psoriasis, there has been a significant effect of obesity in precipitating, aggravating psoriasis as well as reducing the response to treatment in psoriasis.

Key Message

- ***According to this study, there is no significant correlation between the body mass index or waist circumference in the severity of psoriasis.***

ARTICLE 91

Bariatric Surgery and the Incidence of Psoriasis and Psoriatic Arthritis in the Swedish Obese Subjects Study

Maglio C, Peltonen M, Rudin A, et al. Bariatric surgery and the incidence of psoriasis and psoriatic arthritis in the swedish obese subjects study.
Obesity (Silver Spring). 2017;25(12):2068-73.

Abstract

Reduction in body mass index has shown to have a beneficial effect in reduction of severity of psoriasis and also better response. The objective of this study was to find the effect of bariatric surgery on the incidence of psoriasis and psoriatic arthritis. 1991 patients who underwent bariatric surgery and 2018 controls were studied and followed up over a period of 26 years. Bariatric surgery was shown to have a lower risk of development of psoriasis.

COMMENT

This article is a prospective case-control study on the effect of bariatric surgery in obese patients, on the incidence of psoriasis and psoriatic arthritis.

Data were taken from the Swedish National Patient Register and through questionnaires given to the patients. 1991 individuals who underwent bariatric surgery and 2018 obese patients (controls) were taken for the study. These cases and controls were studied over a period of 26 years. The various bariatric surgeries which were performed included gastric bypass, gastric banding and vertical gastroplasty.

A significantly lower incidence of psoriasis was seen in patients who had undergone bariatric surgery as compared to those who had not. Longer duration of psoriasis and smoking both were independently associated with a higher risk of psoriasis. There was no difference in lowering psoriasis incidence risk and the three procedures. However, there was no difference in development of psoriatic arthritis in the control and the surgery groups.

Nicotine could play a role in immune system alteration and skin cell growth, and thus affecting skin inflammation.

Increased body fat is associated with increased levels of inflammatory cytokines which could increase the chance of psoriasis and psoriatic arthritis. Thus, the duration of obesity could be associated with a sustained increase in level of cytokines which will increase the chance of developing psoriasis.

Patients with psoriasis also have unhealthy dietary habits, less exercise (because of lowered self-esteem and body image issues) increased social isolation, depression and alcohol consumption. All these also increase the chances of obesity in psoriasis patients and the patient goes into a vicious cycle of obesity and increase in severity of psoriasis. Moreover, the response of obese psoriasis patients to medication is all less. All these factors make it difficult for an obese psoriasis patient to lose weight.

In this way bariatric surgery may be of help in stopping this vicious cycle of obesity and psoriasis.

Key Message

- ***Bariatric surgery in obese individuals is associated with a lower incidence rate of psoriasis compared with obese individuals who did not undergo the surgery.***

ARTICLE 92

Atorvastatin as Adjunctive Therapy for Chronic Plaque Type Psoriasis versus Betamethasone Valerate Alone: A Randomized, Double-blind, Placebo-controlled Trial

Chua SHH, Tioleco GMS, Dayrit CAF, et al. Atorvastatin as adjunctive therapy for chronic plaque type psoriasis versus betamethasone valerate alone: A randomized, double-blind, placebo-controlled trial.
Indian J Dermatol Venereol Leprol. 2017;83(4):441-7.

Abstract

T helper (Th1) cell mediated chronic inflammation is seen in psoriasis. Stains have an immunomodulatory and anti-inflammatory effects and target Th1 cells. The aim of this study was to examine the safety and efficacy of atorvastatin as an adjunctive treatment for plaque psoriasis. A total of 28 patients were split into two groups one of which received atorvastatin in a dose of 40 mg and the other received a placebo. Both the groups received betamethasone valerate ointment which was applied twice daily for a period of 3 weeks since atorvastatin is technically not a proven treatment for psoriasis. The outcomes studied were reduction in PASI scores and the ratio of patients achieving PASI 50. Atorvastatin helped in reducing PASI scores but did not give an additional benefit to topical steroid application.

COMMENT

This article is a study to evaluate the efficacy of atorvastatin at anti-inflammatory doses in reducing the severity of psoriasis. Statins inhibit 3-hydroxy-3-methyl-glutaryl-coenzyme A reductase and have immunomodulatory and anti-inflammatory effects apart from treatment of dyslipidemia. They inhibit lymphocyte function associated antigen-1 which inhibits the activation and migration of T cells to the skin and thereby reduces the production of interferon-γ, tumor necrosis factor-α and interleukin-1β which are proinflammatory cytokines. All these reduce activation and proliferation of keratinocytes.

This was a randomized, double-blind, placebo-controlled, single center, parallel group trial which was conducted over a period of 9 months in Philippines. A total of 28 patients from the age group of 19–65 years having mild-to-moderate psoriasis with a Psoriasis Area Severity Index (PASI) score of <10 were taken for the trial since it would be unethical to withheld known systemic therapies from patients with moderate-to-severe psoriasis.

The patients were divided into two equal treatment groups by means of a computer-generated randomization table. Fourteen patients received atorvastatin 40 mg once daily and 14 got a similar appearing placebo. All patients were instructed to apply betamethasone valerate 0.1% ointment twice a day for a maximum duration of 3 weeks with a 1-week gap in between throughout the duration of the study.

The parameters which were monitored included percentage reduction of PASI score from baseline (treatment success= at least PASI 50), Dermatology Life Quality Index (DLQI), mean change in high sensitivity C-reactive protein (hsCRP), mean change in lipid profile levels and side effects.

There was a 50% drop out rate due to varying reasons. Both patients from the atorvastatin and placebo showed a good to marked improvement at the end of the study. There was no statistically significant difference in reduction of PASI, hsCRP levels or improvement in DLQI between both the groups. There was significant lower total cholesterol and low-density lipoprotein cholesterol levels in the atorvastatin group compared to the placebo group which was expected.

Adverse effects were seen in two patients and they had liver enzyme elevations and mild muscle aches following 2 days of therapy. Both of these showed spontaneous remission.

Since this is a randomized double-blind control trial, it has the highest value. However, the sample size was very small and moreover with a 50% drop out rate, the validity of the result needs to be reconsidered.

Key Message

- ***Though atorvastatin in a dose of 40 mg is known to have anti-inflammatory effects, in this study there is no additional benefit of atorvastatin in PASI reduction as compared to topical steroids.***

ARTICLE 93

British Association of Dermatologists Guidelines for Biologic Therapy for Psoriasis 2017

Smith CH, Jabbar-Lopez ZK, Yiu ZZ, et al. British association of dermatologists guidelines for biologic therapy for psoriasis 2017.
Br J Dermatol. 2017;177(3):628-36.

Abstract

The aim of this article is to provide a guideline in the use of biologic therapies in psoriasis. Evidence-based recommendations were provided on the use of etanercept, infliximab, adalimumab, secukinumab, ustekinumab and ixekizumab in children, adolescents and adults for the management of psoriasis. These guidelines were developed on the basis of British Association of Dermatologists with Appraisal of Guidelines Research and Evaluation instrument and Grading of Recommendations Assessment, Development and Evaluation as the references.

These guidelines were made for implementation in the National Health Service in the United Kingdom and are for only licenced indications. The guidelines do not cover agents which were licensed out of United Kingdom and do not cover indications except psoriasis or even when the main indication is psoriatic arthritis and not psoriasis.

COMMENT

This article is a set of guidelines devised by the British Association of Dermatologists (BAD) providing evidence-based guidelines for the use of biologic therapies for the treatment of psoriasis and psoriatic arthritis. The biologics studies were adalimumab, etanercept, infliximab, ixekizumab, secukinumab and ustekinumab and the guidelines were applicable to their biosimilars too.

Total 57 recommendations were enumerated in this article, the most important of which will be discussed here.

Biologic therapy is to be offered in psoriasis patients who require systemic therapy when methotrexate and cyclosporin have failed, contraindicated or not tolerated. It is to be started in psoriasis which is an extensive (PASI>10), localized severe disease with significant functional impairment, present in difficult to treat sites or has a significant impact on the quality of life.

The response to biologic therapy is to be reviewed with the improvement in PASI scores (PASI 50 response), control of psoriatic arthritis, improvement in Dermatology Life Quality Index (DLQI) by at least 4 points and adherence to treatment. If there is no minimum response (primary failure), there is initial response but later patient loses response (secondary failure) or if the current biologic therapy is not tolerated, alternative therapy has to be considered which can even be another biologic therapy.

The parameters to be considered before starting on biologic therapy include type of psoriatic arthritis, need of the patient, goal of therapy, disease severity, age, comorbid illness (inflammatory bowel disease or cardiovascular disease), pregnancy plans, weight and adherence of the patient.

The first-line therapy recommended is ustekinumab, secukinumab and adalimumab (especially when psoriatic arthropathy is present). Second line biologics are all the other licensed biologic therapies and they are used when the patient does not respond to first-line therapy. Infliximab is supposed to be reserved for individuals with severe disease and when other biologic agents have failed.

Tumor necrosis factor (TNF) antagonists are supposed to be avoided in patients with demyelinating diseases or when first degree relatives are affected with the demyelinating disease. If any neurological symptoms appear, treatment needs to stopped and specialist advice should be taken. TNF antagonists are supposed to be avoided in patients with cardiac failure too. If the patient has inflammatory bowel disease, a gastroenterologist needs to be consulted before starting the patient on ixekizumab and secukinumab. In case of elective surgery, biologics need to be stopped to prevent postoperative infection.

Key Messages

- ***The first-line therapy recommended is ustekinumab, secukinumab and adalimumab***
- ***Tumor necrosis factor antagonists are to be avoided in case of demyelinating disease in the patient or family and in case of cardiac disease***
- ***Caution should be exerted in giving secukinumab and ixekizumab in case of inflammatory bowel disease.***

ARTICLE 94

Certolizumab Pegol in the Treatment of Psoriasis and Psoriatic Arthritis: Preliminary Real-life Data

Dattola A, Cannizzaro MV, Mazzeo M, et al. Certolizumab pegol in the treatment of psoriasis and psoriatic arthritis: Preliminary real-life data.
Dermatol Ther (Heidelb). 2017;7(4):485-92.

Abstract

Certolizumab Pegol (CZP) is an anti-tumor necrosis factor alpha agent which is approved in Europe for the treatment of psoriatic arthritis and rheumatoid arthritis. A total of 44 patients were studied out of which 41 completed the study. All patients had psoriatic arthritis and 36 had both psoriasis and psoriatic arthritis. CZP showed significant benefits in improvement of the cutaneous and arthritic components of psoriasis with no adverse effects.

COMMENT

This article is a study to evaluate the efficacy of certolizumab pegol (CZP) in the treatment of psoriasis and psoriatic arthritis (PsA).

Certolizumab pegol is a biologic agent which has anti-tumor necrosis factor-alpha properties. It has been used for rheumatoid arthritis and has been FDA approved in 2013 for the treatment of PsA in adults. This drug is given subcutaneously in a dose of 400 mg (two injections of 200 mg) every alternate week for 4 weeks followed by a dose of 200 mg every alternate week.

A total of 44 patients were taken for the study and 41 patients completed the study. Only 32 patients completed 3 months of treatment and 12 patients completed 6 months of treatment. Five patients had only PsA and 36 patients had both psoriasis and PsA. The parameters studies were Psoriasis Area Severity Index (PASI) score, Disease activity score on 44 joints (DASS-44) and a correlation to the ESR (DASS44-ESR).

The efficacy of CZP improved the cutaneous and the arthritis features. There was significant decrease in both the PASI and the DASS44-ESR scores. No adverse effects were seen.

The study was done on a small group of patients and for a short duration of time and moreover no controls were used.

A larger study with more subjects, for a longer follow-up period would be more helpful. A randomized control study model would also be useful.

Key Message

- *Certolizumab pegol is useful in both psoriasis and psoriatic arthritis but more long-term studies are required to further confirm these results.*

ARTICLE 95

Chemerin as a Marker of Subclinical Cardiac Involvement in Psoriatic Patients

Aksu F, Caliskan M, Keles N, et al. Chemerin as a marker of subclinical cardiac involvement in psoriatic patients. *Cardiol J. 2017;24(3):276-83.*

Abstract

Inflammation in psoriasis has been associated with chemerin. The objective of this study was to evaluate whether psoriasis patients with cardiac involvement indicated by impaired flow mediated dilatation, increased epicardial fat tissue and diastolic dysfunction have increased chemerin levels than a healthy control group. A total of 60 patients with psoriasis and 32 healthy controls were studied and the above parameters were studied in all the patients. Psoriasis patients had increased chemerin levels compared to controls. Serum chemerin levels also correlated with the cardiac parameters.

COMMENT

This article is a study on the relationship between the chemerin levels and subclinical cardiac involvement in psoriasis patients.

Psoriasis is associated with early development of atherosclerosis and subclinical left ventricular dysfunction even without presence of any cardiovascular risk factors. This is due to the chronic inflammatory process occurring in psoriasis. Strong chemerin expressions along with increased amount of plasmacytoid dendritic cells have been seen in psoriatic skin. Chemerin is a chemokine which modulates activation and chemotaxis of macrophages, dendritic cells and neutrophils. It is expressed in the liver and adipose tissue and is associated with metabolic syndrome.

A total of 60 psoriatic patients and 32 healthy controls were taken for study. The parameters studied were echocardiographic parameters, flow mediated dilatation, epicardial fat tissue, fasting lipid profile, glucose levels, C-reactive protein levels, body mass index (BMI), waist circumference, Psoriasis Area Severity Index (PASI) score and blood pressure. Chemerin levels were measured with commercial enzyme-linked immunosorbent assay (ELISA) kits.

The chemerin levels in the psoriatic group was higher than the control group. All the diastolic function parameters were impaired in the psoriasis patient group. Epicardial fat was more in the psoriatic patients. There was a positive correlation between chemerin levels and the age, blood pressure, waist circumference and BMI.

This study was done in a small group of patients. A larger study with equal number of patients and controls will be useful in further confirming the findings of this study.

Key Messages

- ***There is a significant relationship between chemerin levels and the epicardial fat thickness and flow mediated dilatation which are both signs of subclinical atherosclerosis. It is also a marker of diastolic function***
- ***Chemerin can be used as a marker to screen patients for subclinical cardiac disease.***

ARTICLE 96

Clinical Efficacy and IL-17 Targeting Mechanism of *Indigo naturalis* as a Topical Agent in Moderate Psoriasis

Cheng HM, Wu YC, Wang Q, et al. Clinical efficacy and IL-17 targeting mechanism of Indigo naturalis as a topical agent in moderate psoriasis.
BMC Complement Altern Med. 2017;17:439.

Abstract

Indigo naturalis is a native Chinese medicine which is used for many inflammatory disorders including psoriasis. A randomized double-blind placebo-controlled trial using *Indigo naturalis* topically showed significant improvement in PASI scores as compared to controls. This study also examined the effect of *Indigo naturalis* on *in vitro* keratinocytes and found out that tryptanthrin, a component of *Indigo naturalis* has an IL-17 inhibitory effect.

COMMENT

This article is a study on the clinical efficacy of *Indigo naturalis* as a topical monotherapy to treat mild-to-moderate psoriasis.

This was a randomized placebo-controlled study in which double-blind was conducted with a total of 24 patients among which 16 were treated with *Indigo naturalis* ointment and 8 with placebo twice daily for 8 weeks with follow-ups at 1-week intervals.

A global gene expression analysis of affected skin was also conducted to find out a molecular signature of moderate psoriasis and the impact of *Indigo naturalis* treatment on it. Chemical components of *Indigo naturalis* were also evaluated for anti-IL-17 induced cytokine release in cultured keratinocytes.

Topicals are generally used as first-line agents to treat mild-to-moderate psoriasis. However, long-term use of topical steroids is associated with side effects. Topical traditional Chinese medicines with a key compound being *Indigo naturalis* have been commonly used in alternate therapies in the Asia Pacific region.

Indigo naturalis is a dried pigment prepared from several plant species including *Baphicacanthus cusia*. Indirubin, a component of *Indigo naturalis* has been reported to inhibit signal transducer and activator of transcription-3 (STAT3) activities, cyclin dependant kinase and keratinocyte proliferation *in vitro*. Tryptanthrin, another component has been reported to inhibit interferon-γ production by lymphocytes and prostaglandin E2 synthesis and nitric oxide synthesis in murine macrophages. It also inhibits oxygen generation and elastase release in human neutrophils.

The *Indigo naturalis* ointment used in the study has a ration of 1:10 of *Indigo naturalis* powder and a vehicle containing olive oil: microcrystalline wax: Vaseline in a ratio of 9:6:5. There was a significant improvement in the Psoriasis Area Severity Index (PASI) score at 8 weeks of treatment with 56.3% patients showing PASI 75 compared with 0% in placebo.

A gene expression study from baseline skin biopsies established upregulation of interleukin-17 as a key component in psoriasis. Treatment with *Indigo naturalis* resulting in down-regulation of IL-17 pathway especially with the tryptanthrin component (established through an *in vitro* study).

Key Messages

- *Indigo naturalis showed good clinical efficacy in mild-to-moderate psoriasis with significant reduction of PASI scores compared to controls*
- *The mechanism of action of Indigo naturalis is down-regulation of IL-17 pathway.*

ARTICLE 97

Comparative Evaluation of Efficacy and Safety of Calcipotriol versus Tacalcitol Ointment, Both in Combination with NBUVB Phototherapy in the Treatment of Stable Plaque Psoriasis

Dua I, Aggarwal K, Jian VK. Comparative evaluation of efficacy and safety of calcipotriol versus tacalcitol ointment, both in combination with NBUVB phototherapy in the treatment of stable plaque psoriasis.
Photodermatol Photoimmunol Photomed. 2017;33(5):275-81.

Abstract

Both vitamin D analogues and NBUVB phototherapy are established modalities for the treatment of psoriasis. The aim of this study was to compare calcipotriol and tacalcitol both in combination with NBUVB phototherapy in the treatment of chronic plaque psoriasis. The left side was treated with tacalcitol and right side with calcipotriol topically. Both sides were given NBUVB therapy thrice weekly. Target plaque scoring was used to assess efficacy. Both the vitamin D analogues were effective and safe but calcipotriol was more effective with a faster onset of action and better response maintenance.

COMMENT

This article is a study to compare the safety and efficacy of two vitamin D analogues, tacalcitol and calcipotriol along with narrow-band ultraviolet B (NB-UVB) therapy in the treatment of psoriasis.

Vitamin D analogs act by binding to the intracellular vitamin D receptor which subsequently binds to and regulates the genes which are involved in inflammation, epidermal proliferation and keratinization. Synthetic vitamin D analogs have been developed by modification of the side chain which increases the anti-psoriatic effect and it is rapidly transformed into inactive metabolites which decrease the hypercalcemic action.

In this study, 30 patients were studied over a period of 12 weeks. Left side was treated with tacalcitol ointment once daily and the right side with calcipotriol ointment twice daily. Narrow-band UVB was give thrice weekly. Target plaque scoring was used to assess efficacy.

There was significant improvement in target plaque severity score with significant reduction of scaling, erythema and induration with both topicals with improvement starting at 2 weeks of therapy. There was rapid clearance of plaques in both groups. However, there were relapses which were less so with calcipotriol. Moreover, the number of sessions and the cumulative NB-UVB dose was lower in the calcipotriol group.

Thus, calcipotriol ointments can be combined with NB-UVB therapy for treatment of plaque psoriasis. By reducing the cumulative amount of NB-UVB required; it can help in reducing the side effects of NB-UVB.

A larger randomized control study with even tacalcitol being used twice daily will help in cementing the results of this study.

Key Messages

- ***Both tacalcitol and calcipotriol topical applications in combination with NB-UVB help in reducing the target plaque score***
- ***Calcipotriol has more efficacy, faster onset of action, is better tolerated and has a better maintenance of response than tacalcitol.***

ARTICLE 98

Comparison of Ixekizumab with Ustekinumab in Moderate-to-Severe Psoriasis: 24-Week Results from IXORA-S, a Phase III Study

Reich K, Pinter A, Lacour JP, et al. Comparison of ixekizumab with ustekinumab in moderate-to-severe psoriasis: 24-week results from IXORA-S, a phase III study.
Br J Dermatol. 2017;177(4):1014-23.

Abstract

Interleukin-23 and interleukin-17 axis is of utmost importance in psoriasis pathogenesis. The objective of this study was to compare the safety and efficacy of ixekizumab versus ustekinumab. The patients were examined at week 12 and week 24. The parameters taken into consideration were PASI 90, PASI 75, PASI 100, Physicians Global Assessment score of 0 or 1, DLQI of 0 and more than 4-point reduction of numerical rating scale and changes in skin pain visual analogue scale. Ixekizumab showed superior efficacy which was demonstrated at 12 weeks and persisted till week 24. Neither of the treatments had any significant adverse effects.

COMMENT

This article is a study on the comparison of ixekizumab (IXE) with ustekinumab (UST) in the treatment of moderate-to-severe psoriasis.

This was a randomized phase III study conducted over a period of 24 weeks. The patients were evaluated at the end of week 12 and week 24. A total of 136 patients received IXE in a dose of 160 mg starting dose subcutaneously followed by 80 mg every 2 weeks for 12 weeks and then subsequently 80 mg every 4 weeks. About 166 patients received USR in a dose of 45 mg or 90 mg according to their body weight.

The proportion of patients reaching PASI 90 (90% or more improvement in Psoriasis Area Severity Index) was calculated. The various endpoints taken into consideration were PASI 75, PASI 100, sPGA (static Physician's Global Assessment score of 0 or 1), DLQI (Dermatology Life Quality Index) of 0 or 1, 4 or more-point reduction in the itch numerical rating scale (NRS) and changes in the skin pain visual analogue scale and the itch NRS.

Ixekizumab is humanized monoclonal immunoglobulin G and is one of the three biologic agents (the other two being brodalumab and secukinumab) which targets the interleukin-17 (IL-17) cytokine pathway. Interleukin-17 plays a role in activation and recruitment of neutrophils, prevents neutrophil apoptosis and stimulates angiogenesis in psoriasis. Interleukin-17A is one of the six homodimers of IL-17 and is the most potent isoform implicated in development of psoriasis. Ixekizumab specifically binds to and inhibits IL-17A and prevents the inflammatory changes which lead to psoriasis. Ustekinumab is a human monoclonal antibody which targets the p40 subunit shared by two cytokines namely IL-12 and IL-23 which prevents their interaction with the receptor and thus prevents the signaling, differentiation and cytokine production in inflammatory diseases such as psoriasis.

At the end of 12 weeks IXE showed better response in terms of PASI 90, PASI 75, PASI 100 and sPGA. At the end of week 24, IXE showed significantly better results in all the above parameters as well as in DLQI.

The adverse effects reported were not significant enough to halt treatment and no deaths were reported. The adverse effect incidence did not vary significantly between the two biologics.

Phase IV post marketing surveillance will also have to be done to see the long-term side effects and benefits of IXE.

Key Message

- ***Ixekizumab demonstrated better efficacy than ustekinumab in the treatment of moderate-to-severe plaque psoriasis with respect to PASI 90, PASI 75, PASI 100, improvement in sPGA and DLQI at both 12 weeks and 24 weeks of treatment.***

ARTICLE 99

Comparison of Phenotype, Comorbidities, Therapy and Adverse Events between Psoriatic Patients with and without Psoriatic Arthritis. Biobadaderm Registry

Pérez-Plaza A, Carretero G, Ferrandiz C, et al. Comparison of phenotype, comorbidities, therapy and adverse events between psoriatic patients with and without psoriatic arthritis. Biobadaderm registry.
J Eur Acad Dermatol Venereol. 2017;31(6):1021-8.

Abstract

The number of studies comparing psoriasis patients with and without arthritis are limited. The objective of this study was to compare the phenotype, therapeutic profile, baseline comorbidities and incidence of adverse effects in psoriasis patients with and without psoriatic arthritis. The patients were selected from the Biobadaderm registry and patients were divided into two groups namely psoriasis without arthritis and psoriasis with psoriatic arthritis (PsA). The patients were followed up and monitored for any joint involvement. A total of 2,120 patients were taken among which 1,871 had psoriasis without PsA and 249 had psoriasis and PsA. The patients with PsA had significantly more comorbidities such as liver disease, hypertension, used more systemic therapies especially combination therapy and anti-TNF-α drugs and had more adverse effects including more serious adverse effects. This indicates that patients with both psoriasis and PsA should be managed and followed up more closely.

COMMENT

This article is a comparative analysis on the comorbidities, therapeutic prolife, phenotype and adverse effects such as infections, infestations, psychiatric disorders and malignancies in psoriatic patients with and without arthritis.

This was a prospective cohort analysis. Data were collected from the Biobadaderm registry. The patients were split into two groups at the time of entry into the analysis: Those with psoriasis without arthritis and psoriasis patients with psoriatic arthritis (PsA). Since PsA may develop later also and has a positive correlation with the duration of the disease, patients who developed signs or symptoms of joint involvement later during follow-up in the first group were excluded from the analysis.

A total of 2,120 patients were analyzed of which 1,870 patients had psoriasis without PsA and 249 patients had both psoriasis and PsA. It was found out that the patients with PsA had more comorbidities including liver disease, hypertension; they used a larger amount of systemic medication such as combination therapy and biologics and had more adverse effects and serious adverse effects. The rate of infections and infestations was also more in the PsA group.

Psoriatic arthritis itself is considered to be a complication of psoriasis and the incidence of which increases with the increased duration of the disease. It does not have a relation with the Psoriasis Area Severity Index (PASI) or Nail Psoriasis Severity Index (NAPSI) scores which means even with less extensive skin lesions, the patient can have a more severe joint involvement.

With increased duration of psoriasis, the complications and risk of metabolic syndrome, other inflammatory conditions and infections increases. Therefore, it is expected that PsA which usually occurs in the later period of psoriasis, should be associated with more complications that if the patient had only psoriasis without PsA.

Single nucleotide polymorphisms in the IL-13 gene have to be associated with specific risk of PsA. There is higher incidence of PsA in obese or overweight individuals compared to normal weight patients with psoriasis. Infections such as *Streptococcus* and human immunodeficiency virus (HIV), joint trauma and emotional stress act as a trigger for PsA.

Moll and wright criteria, Psoriatic arthritis screening and evaluation (PASE) score and Classification of Psoriatic Arthritis (CASPAR) study group criteria can be used to diagnose PsA.

Key Messages

- *There are more comorbidities and complications associated with patients having both PsA and psoriasis that in patients with psoriasis without PsA*
- *Therefore, patients with psoriasis and PsA should be more carefully monitored.*

ARTICLE 100

Depression and Suicidality in Psoriasis: Review of the Literature Including the Cytokine Theory of Depression

Koo J, Marangell LB, Nakamura M, et al. Depression and suicidality in psoriasis: Review of the literature including the cytokine theory of depression.
J Eur Acad Dermatol Venereol. 2017;31(12):1999-2009.

Abstract

Psoriasis has a lot of physical symptoms and patients feel a lot of stigma due to the appearance of their skin. Depression, anxiety and suicidal tendencies are widely prevalent in psoriasis patients. Apart from severe cutaneous disease leading to psychiatric comorbidities, there is a common biological mechanism in both psoriasis and depression. There is elevation of proinflammatory cytokines such as IL-6 and IL-1 in both depression and psoriasis. This is a review of literature which analyzed the mechanism by which elevated cytokines and inflammatory response leads to depression. Systemic inflammation which is seen in psoriasis plays a role in mental comorbidities such as depression and suicidal ideation and behavior.

COMMENT

This article is a review of literature on depression and suicidal tendencies in psoriasis. It also reviewed the cytokine theory of depression in inflammatory disorders.

Psoriasis patients feel a stigma due to the appearance of their skin and are also socially isolated. Anxiety, suicidal ideation and behavior (SIB), and depression along with other mental health comorbidities are commonly seen in patients with psoriasis. The degree of the disorder also varies with the severity of the disease. Since both psoriasis and psychiatric conditions progress with aggravation of either one of these conditions, they may have similar biological mechanisms. IL-1 and IL-6 which are both proinflammatory cytokines which are increased in both these conditions.

Cytokine level elevation in the central nervous system can lead to certain biochemical changes which can lead to depression. Brain-derived neurotrophic factor (BNDF), a neurotrophin which plays a key role in mental disorders was reduced in both depression and psoriasis. Type-1 cell activity is implicated in the pathogenesis of depression (major depressive disorder has immune system dysregulation and increased levels of CXCL10/IP-10) which is also seen implicated in psoriasis. High levels of proinflammatory cytokines like IL-6 and tumor necrosis factor-α (TNF-α) has been seen in depressed patients who do not have other pre-existing chronic inflammatory disorder. Administration of interferon-α which is a proinflammatory cytokine leads to depression in half of depressive patients in a study.

Decreased melatonin levels are seen both in psoriasis and depression. There is increased percentage of CD2+, CD4+ and CD8+ lymphocytes and reduced percentage of CD4+

lymphocytes in both psoriasis and depression. Increased levels of peripheral inflammatory biomarkers including inflammatory cytokines are elevated in both the conditions.

Key Messages

- *Apart from the negative psychological effects which are present in any skin disorder with or without inflammation such as low self-esteem and social anxiety leading to depression, the inflammatory cytokines released in psoriasis are those which are also released in depression*
- *Therefore, psoriasis and depression have a predisposition to aggravate the other condition since the cytokines released in both the conditions are same*
- *Hence a dermatologist, psychiatrist and psychologist should work in tandem to manage a case of psoriasis associated with depression*
- *If a psoriasis patient already has a depressive disorder prior to developing psoriasis, extra care must be taken.*

ARTICLE 101

Development of Paradoxical Inflammatory Disorders During Treatment of Psoriasis with TNF Inhibitors: A Review of Published Cases

Havmose M, Thomsen SF. Development of paradoxical inflammatory disorders during treatment of psoriasis with TNF inhibitors: A review of published cases.
Int J Dermatol. 2017;56(11):1087-1102.

Abstract

Tumor necrosis factor inhibitors have been used effectively in the treatment of psoriasis. Infections and malignancies are established side effects whereas certain paradoxical non-neoplastic non-infectious inflammatory side effects are less recognized. The aim of the study was the identification of published paradoxical inflammatory adverse effects which are non-infectious and non-neoplastic in patients of psoriasis on TNF inhibitors. The search was done in MEDLINE and a total of 269 patients were identified to develop this adverse effect to etanercept (101), adalimumab (102) and infliximab (91). One case report was related to both etanercept and adalimumab. The large number of cases having this side effect indicates the need for surveillance of patients on TNF inhibitor therapy.

COMMENT

This article is a review of paradoxical inflammatory disorders seen with tumor necrosis factor-α (TNF-α) inhibitors which are non-infectious and non-neoplastic.

Tumor necrosis factor-α inhibitors are considered to be relatively safe and effective in the management of psoriasis. The commonly used TNF-α inhibitors in psoriasis include etanercept, infliximab and adalimumab. All three block TNF-α *in vivo*, but differ in structure and mechanism of action. Infliximab is a chimeric human/ murine monoclonal antibody which binds to both membrane bound and soluble TNF-α, and neutralizes its action. Adalimumab is a full human antibody which has similar mechanism of action as infliximab. Etanercept is a receptor fusion protein which has two human TNF-α receptors fused to the Fc portion of the human antibody. Etanercept binds to free TNF-α and thus weakly inhibits TNF-α trimers *in vivo*. Infliximab since it is nonhuman (chimeric), it has higher risk of inducing neutralizing antibodies especially in patients on intermittent treatment.

A paradoxical reaction is one when there is either onset or exacerbation of a symptom or disease following the administration of a medicine which has been proven to be efficacious for the same condition.

The paradoxical reactions to TNF-α inhibitors include cutaneous, digestive, arthropathic and ophthalmic conditions. The paradoxical reactions include psoriasis, psoriatic arthritis, hidradenitis suppurativa and inflammatory bowel diseases like Crohn's disease, uveitis, sarcoidosis, granulomatous disorders, vasculitis and alopecia areata. The hypotheses to explain these reactions include an imbalance in cytokine production, unopposed type I interferon production, shift towards Th1/ Th2 profile and differential immunological properties between monoclonal antibodies and TNF-α soluble receptor.

Literature search was performed using MEDLINE. A total of 295 cases were studied from 13 articles. Only 265 cases had a paradoxical adverse effect (PAE); 91, 101 and 102 cases were linked to infliximab, etanercept and adalimumab respectively. One report was related to both adalimumab and etanercept.

The large numbers of PAE which are non-neoplastic and non-infective suggest that continuous surveillance of patients who are on TNF-α inhibitors for psoriasis is necessary.

Key Messages

- *A large number of patients develop paradoxical inflammatory effect to TNF-a inhibitors which are non-infectious and non-neoplastic*
- *These inflammatory reactions may be cutaneous, digestive, ophthalmic or digestive conditions*
- *Constant monitoring of patients on TNF-a inhibitors is necessary to detect these paradoxical adverse effects.*

ARTICLE 102

Effects of Wannachawee Recipe with Antipsoriatic Activity on Suppressing Inflammatory Cytokine Production in HaCaT Human Keratinocytes

Na Takuathung M, Wongnoppavich A, Pitchakarn P, et al. Effects of Wannachawee recipe with antipsoriatic activity on suppressing inflammatory cytokine production in HaCaT human keratinocytes.
Evid Based Complement Alternat Med. 2017;2017:5906539.

Abstract

Psoriasis is an immune mediated chronic inflammatory disease. T cell activation is present through the IL-23/Th17 axis. Conventional modalities of treatment are associated with adverse effects which in turn has an effect on the patient's adherence to treatment. Wannachawee Recipe (WCR) is a Thai folk remedy used for the treatment of psoriasis. The aim of this study was to define the mechanism of anti-inflammatory and anti-proliferation effects of WCR in HaCaT cells.

COMMENT

This article is a study on the effect of Wannachawee recipe (WCR) on HaCaT human keratinocytes. It assessed the suppression of inflammatory cytokine production and inhibition of cell cycle.

Wannachawee recipe is a Thai traditional medicine which used different plants and has been enlisted in the Hospital Traditional Medicine Formulary. The components in WCR are *Alpinia galanga, Smilax glabra, Smilax corbularia, Stemona involuta, Smilax glabra, Rhinacanthus nasutus* and *Acanthus ilicifolius.*

A previous study was done on WCR in 136 psoriasis patients who were given 10.77 g of WCR per day for a period of 6–7 months and the psoriasis severity was compared. Approximately, 93% patients had good response with WCR.

The factors which aggravated psoriasis included stress, sleep deprivation, chemical and ultraviolet light exposure and a particular diet. This study was aimed at investigating the mechanism for the therapeutic effect of WCR specifically on the anti-inflammatory and anti-proliferation potential on HaCaT keratinocytes. The HaCaT keratinocytes are immortalized human epidermal keratinocytes which have high rates of proliferation. Acitretin and methotrexate were used as positive controls.

Wannachawee recipe inhibited the growth and viability of HaCaT cells in a concentration dependent manner, but did not have an effect on the cell cycle progression. It decreased the mRNA expression of many inflammatory factors such as IL-23, IL-17A, IL-6, IL-1β, IL-8 and tumor necrosis factor-α (TNF-α). Thus, WCR has an anti-inflammatory effect without having cellular toxicity and thus is effective in psoriasis therapy.

In the previous study, WCR had showed good clinical effect and in this study beneficial effects were seen *in vitro*.

Key Messages

- *Wannachawee recipe is a Thai traditional medicine which has anti-inflammatory benefits and decreases expression and production of inflammatory cytokines which are involved in the pathogenesis of psoriasis but does not have effect on cell cycle progression*
- *It has also shown good clinical benefit by decreasing the severity in psoriasis patients when given for a period of 6–7 months.*

ARTICLE 103

Effectiveness of Lipid-lowering Statin Therapy in Patients with and without Psoriasis

Ports WC, Fayyad R, DeMicco DA, et al. Effectiveness of lipid-lowering statin therapy in patients with and without psoriasis.
Clin Drug Investig. 2017;37(8):775-85.

Abstract

Psoriasis has been associated with metabolic syndrome and dyslipidemia which is associated with cardiovascular risk. This study compared the effects of statin therapy on cardiovascular outcomes and lipid levels in patients with and without psoriasis. One primary, two secondary cardiovascular prevention statin trials and IDEAL trial were analyzed. The parameters studied were cardiovascular event rates, baseline characteristics and lipid changes from baseline. Improved cardiovascular outcomes and improved lipid levels with statin therapy was seen in patients with and without psoriasis supporting the use of statins in psoriasis.

COMMENT

This article is an analysis on the use of statin therapy in patients with and without psoriasis.

Psoriasis patients have increased prevalence of atherosclerotic disease such as cerebrovascular disease, coronary artery disease and peripheral vascular disease, and also have an increased risk of myocardial infraction. Inflammation may be a linking factor in both the diseases.

Statins are reversible competitive inhibitors of 3-hydroxyl-3-methylyglutaryl-coenzyme A reductase, a rare limiting enzyme in cholesterol biosynthesis. Statins also have anti-inflammatory effect and help to reduce atherogenesis and thus cardiovascular morbidity. It helps to reduce the release of C-reactive proteins, cytokines, chemokines and adhesion molecules, and modulates T cell activity which will also help to reduce the inflammatory component of psoriasis.

Psoriasis by itself is and independent risk factor for cardiovascular disease as a result of systemic inflammation and aggravation of atherosclerosis. Psoriasis and atherosclerosis have a lot of similar pathogenic mechanisms such as both being Th1 mediated, both having same pattern of T cell activation and adhesion molecule expression and both having involvement of monocytes, macrophages, T cells, extracellular matrix and connective tissue cells.

Statins down regulate adhesion molecules such as LFA-1 (target of efalizumab), inhibit production of inflammatory cytokines like TNF-α (target of adalimumab, infliximab and etanercept), inhibit production of IL-17 (target of secukinumab) and inhibit activation and migration of Th1 cells.

This analysis assessed patients from one primary and two secondary cardiovascular prevention statin trials. The parameters taken into consideration were baseline characteristics, cardiovascular changes and lipid changes from baseline.

The lipid profile improvement with statins was similar in patients with and without psoriasis. High dose atorvastatin was significantly more effective in reducing cardiovascular events than low dose statin therapy.

Key Messages

- ***Psoriasis and atherosclerosis have similar pathogenic mechanisms related to inflammation***
- ***The improvement in lipid levels with statins was similar in patients with and without psoriasis***
- ***High dose statin therapy significantly reduced the risk of cardiovascular events in psoriasis patients.***

ARTICLE 104

Effects of Nanoparticles with Hydrotropic Nicotinamide on Tacrolimus: Permeability through Psoriatic Skin and Antipsoriatic and Antiproliferative Activities

Wan T, Pan W, Long Y, et al. Effects of nanoparticles with hydrotropic nicotinamide on tacrolimus: Permeability through psoriatic skin and antipsoriatic and antiproliferative activities.
Int J Nanomedicine. 2017;12:1485-97.

Abstract

A hybrid system composed of nanoparticles made by the combination of hyaluronic acid with cholesterol along with nicotinamide and tacrolimus has proven to have a synergistic effect on the penetration of tacrolimus into intact skin. The aim of this study was to study the potential of this combination for the treatment of psoriasis. The antipsoriatic effect of this combination was studied for imiquimod induced psoriasis. The results of this combination were comparable to that achieved by clobetasol propionate and better than commercial tacrolimus ointment. Histologically, there was synergistic effect of this combination against psoriasis. This combination also had an anti-proliferative effect on HaCaT cell proliferation.

COMMENT

This article is a study on the use of nano-particles (NPs) made by the combination of hyaluronic acid and cholesterol in combination with nicotinic acid for the penetration of tacrolimus into intact skin. This will help to evaluate the potential of this combination for psoriasis.

This combination of FK-506 NP-NIC (Tacrolimus, nanoparticles, nicotinamide) had a better effect on the penetration of tacrolimus into intact skin. *In-vitro* tests were carried out on the penetration of this combination on imiquimod induced psoriatic skin and it had a better effect on penetration of tacrolimus through psoriatic skin and also deposition in psoriatic skin.

The Psoriasis Area Severity Index (PASI) score reduction with both FK-506 NP-NIC was similar to that of clobetasol propionate and was significantly more than the commercially available tacrolimus ointment.

On histological examination, there was a synergistic effect of tacrolimus, nicotinamide and NP. Since there is a synergistic effect, less dose of tacrolimus will be required for the same therapeutic effect with less systemic toxicity.

HaCaT is an aneuploid immortal keratinocyte cell line from adult human skin which is spontaneously transformed. It is used in scientific research since it has high ability to differentiate and proliferate *in vitro*. This helps to overcome issues such as short culture life span and variations between cell lines.

The FK-506 NP-NIC combination had significant inhibitory effect on the proliferation of HaCaT and thus will be helpful in psoriasis.

This is mainly an *in vitro* study. An *in vivo* study on psoriasis patients is required to confirm the findings in this study.

If confirmed, it could help to reduce the side effects of long-term topical corticosteroids.

Key Messages

- ***Nanoparticles made of hyaluronic acid and cholesterol in combination with nicotinic acid helps in better penetration and better deposition of tacrolimus into psoriatic skin***
- ***It also has a synergistic effect and has a PASI reduction effect comparable to clobetasol propionate***
- ***This combination also inhibits proliferation of HaCaT lines.***

ARTICLE 105

Guselkumab for the Treatment of Psoriasis: A Review of Phase III Trials

Nakamura M, Lee K, Jeon C, et al. Guselkumab for the treatment of psoriasis: A review of phase III trials. ***Dermatol Ther (Heidelb). 2017;7(3):281-292.***

Abstract

Interleukin-23 (IL-23) inhibitors (guselkumab) are recently used biologics in treatment of psoriasis.

To demonstrate the efficacy and safety of guselkumab in psoriatic patients, the study utilizes data from VOYAGE 1 and VOYAGE 2 trials. At week 16, the proportion of patients attaining at least a 90% improvement from baseline in the Psoriasis Area and Severity Index (PASI 90) was 73.3% in VOYAGE 1 and 70.0% in VOYAGE 2. Guselkumab stayed efficacious up to 48 weeks of treatment. Adverse events like nasopharyngitis, headache, and upper respiratory tract infection are noted.

Phase III trials of guselkumab suggest a constructive efficacy and safety profile of this novel drug. Future studies are required, to evaluate the safety and efficacy for longer period. Still, guselkumab appears to be a potential therapeutic option for psoriasis.

COMMENT

Psoriasis is a common, chronic, immune-mediated skin disease that is painful, disfiguring, and disabling, thereby negatively impacting health-related quality of life (HRQoL) to a significant extent. Psoriasis affecting the body regions such as the scalp, nails, palms and soles are particularly challenging to treat. Elucidation of the pathogenesis of psoriasis has led to effective biologic treatments targeting tumor necrosis factor-alpha (TNF-α), both interleukin (IL)-12 and IL-23 and most recently IL-17 and IL-23, alone.

Guselkumab is a fully human IgG1 lambda monoclonal antibody that binds to the p19 subunit of IL-23 and inhibits the intracellular and downstream signaling of IL-23, which is required for terminal differentiation and survival of T helper (Th) 17 cells. The onset of action of guselkumab was rapid, with significant response as early as 2 week compared with placebo.

The study utilizes data from VOYAGE 1 and VOYAGE 2 trials. Psoriasis Area Severity Index (PASI) 90 and PASI 75 response was high in guselkumab compared to placebo. Psoriatic patients who failed to adalimumab responded to guselkumab. Even after stopping guselkumab, it takes 15.2 weeks for PASI 90 to reduce. PASI 90 in more than 70% by guselkumab gives a remarkable impact on patient's quality of life.

On whole guselkumab seems to have a safety profile. The most common adverse effects seen are nasopharyngitis and upper respiratory tract infection. Serious infection and malignancy are not reported in guselkumab compared to adalimumab and placebo.

Further long-term studies are warranted to validate the promising long-term efficacy and safety profile of guselkumab.

Key Message

- ***Guselkumab is superior to placebo at week 16 and is better able to clear or almost clear psoriasis plaques compared to adalimumab.***

ARTICLE 106

Effectiveness and Safety of Secukinumab in 69 Patients with Moderate to Severe Plaque Psoriasis: A Retrospective Multicenter Study

Schwensen JF, Clemmensen A, Sand C, et al. Effectiveness and safety of secukinumab in 69 patients with moderate to severe plaque psoriasis: A retrospective multicenter study.
Dermatol Ther. 2017;30(6):e12550.

Abstract

Secukinumab is an IL-17A inhibitor which is useful in the treatment of moderate-to-severe plaque psoriasis. In this study 69 Danish patients studied with secukinumab were also studied to assess their safety and efficacy. Majority of the patients in this study were previously refractory to other biologic treatment. The percentage of patients achieving a PASI 50 and 75 at week 12 were recorded. The adverse effect profile was also studied. Secukinumab seems to be an effective treatment modality in patients of moderate-to-severe plaque psoriasis who were not responding or have side effects to traditional biologic agents.

COMMENT

This article is a retrospective multi-center study on the safety and efficacy of secukinumab in patients with moderate-to-severe psoriasis.

Secukinumab is the first IL-17A inhibitor which is approved for the treatment of moderate-to-severe psoriasis in adult patients. Interleukin-17A is important in the pathogenesis of psoriasis and Th17/IL-17 axis dysfunction is an important cause for inflammation. The principal effector cytokine of Th17 cells is IL-17A which stimulates keratinocytes to produce cytokines, chemokines and other proinflammatory mediators which helps to sustain chronic inflammation. Thus, inhibition of IL-17 signaling helps to disrupt the psoriatic inflammatory loop.

Secukinumab is given subcutaneously in a dose of 300 mg (two injections of 150 mg) as the first dose. Following the first dose weekly injections are given for four weeks followed by monthly injections.

Most of the side effects are minor and include redness, swelling and bruising at the injection site. Other side effects include upper respiratory tract infection, nasopharyngitis, rhinitis, candidiasis, urticaria, diarrhea, headache, and arthralgia. Some of the serious side effects include severe infections like tuberculosis and hepatitis. It can also cause a flare-up of Crohn's disease.

In this study 69 Danish patients treated with secukinumab were studied. Approximately, 92.8% of these patients were refractory to other biologic treatment. The initial median Psoriasis Area Severity Index (PASI) score was 7.1. The PASI 50 and PASI 75 achievement at the end of 12 weeks were 66.7% and 52.9% respectively. A PASI score of <2 and <5 were achieved by 60.4% and 83% patients respectively. One-third of the patients stopped treatment due to less improvement and side effects within a period of 51–212 days. A total of 18 patients had side effects.

A study with larger group of patients is necessary to confirm the findings. Moreover, most of the patients studied were resistant to other biologic treatment. A direct comparative study preferably a randomized double-blind study with secukinumab comparing it with other biologics on patients who were not treated with biologics is necessary.

Key Messages

- ***Secukinumab is an effective treatment option in patients with moderate-to-severe plaque psoriasis especially in patients who are refractory to other biologic therapies***
- ***Long-term studies are required to assess the remission rates and long-term side effect profile on treatment with secukinumab.***

ARTICLE 107

Diagnosis and Management of Psoriasis

Kim WB, Jerome D, Yeung J. Diagnosis and management of psoriasis.
Can Fam Physician. 2017;63(4):278-85.

Abstract

The objective of this review was to provide advice on the diagnosis and management of psoriasis. Various databases such as PubMed, EMBASE, MEDLINE and Cochrane were searched for various randomized controlled trials, meta-analyses, observational studies and systematic reviews. Most patients go for initial diagnosis and management to their respective primary healthcare providers. Therefore, it is important to recognize psoriasis and also its medical and psychiatric impact which will help in its proper diagnosis and treatment. Milder cases can be managed with topical therapies, whereas more severe and refractory cases need to be referred to dermatologists for evaluation and systemic therapy.

COMMENT

The article is an overview on the diagnosis and management of psoriasis. Data were collected from PubMed, EMBASE, Cochrane, and MEDLINE databases. Various types of articles were reviewed which included-observational studies, systematic reviews, meta-analyses and randomized controlled trials.

Psoriasis is an inflammatory disease in which there is involvement of multiple systems predominantly the skin, and joint involvement. There is a bimodal age of onset; 16–22 and 57–60 years. Gender incidence is equal.

It has a multifactorial pathogenesis having unrelated inflammation and genetic associations. It has an emotional and psychosocial effect on patients which can result in poor self-esteem, increased stress and poor self-esteem which can affect relationships and social functioning.

Psoriasis is mainly diagnosed clinically. The most common type of psoriasis is chronic plaque psoriasis. The other variants include pustular, inverse, guttate, erythrodermic and annular psoriasis.

The severity of the disease is classified as mild, moderate and severe. Mild psoriasis involves <3% of body surface area (BSA), had minimal effect on the Quality of Life (QoL) and can achieve good results with routine skin care measures and topical treatment. Moderate psoriasis involves 3-10% of BSA, substantially affects the QoL and cannot be only controlled with routine skin care measures. Severe psoriasis involves more than 10% of BSA, causes severe degradation of QoL and cannot expect to be controlled by topical therapy.

Topical therapy includes corticosteroids, calcipotriol and a combination of both. Psoralen and ultraviolet A (PUVA) and ultraviolet B (UVB) phototherapy can be given either in combination with methotrexate and acitretin. First-line non-biologic therapy includes methotrexate, cyclosporine, acitretin and apremilast and biologic therapy includes adalimumab, etanercept, secukinumab, infliximab, and ustekinumab. Second-line therapy includes methotrexate, acitretin or UVB in combination with biologics. This article suggests that patients with mild psoriasis can be treated with topicals by primary healthcare physicians whereas patients with more severe disease require evaluation and management by dermatologists.

Key Messages

- ***Psoriasis is a multisystem chronic inflammatory disorder which is not properly diagnosed and treated despite having a wide prevalence and effect on QoL***
- ***Psoriasis affects mainly the skin and the joints but also has a lot of medical and psychological co-morbidities including diabetes, cardiovascular disease, malignancy as well as anxiety and depression***
- ***The diagnosis is mainly clinical and severity of the disease decides the treatment.***

ARTICLE 108

Early Relapse of Psoriasis after Stopping Brodalumab: A Retrospective Cohort Study in 77 Patients

Masson Regnault M, Konstantinou MP, Khemis A, et al. Early relapse of psoriasis after stopping brodalumab: A retrospective cohort study in 77 patients.
J Eur Acad Dermatol Venereol. 2017;31(9):1491-6.

Abstract

Biologics which target IL-17 have been effective in the treatment and clearing lesions in moderate-to-severe psoriasis. The objective of this study was to analyze the pattern of recurrence of psoriasis following cessation of brodalumab. This was subsequent to Amgen stopping the clinical program in June 2015. Relapse was considered when the patient requested a new treatment following withdrawal of brodalumab. A total of 77 patients were followed up. At the time of cessation 67 of the patients had achieved PASI 90. All the 77 patients relapsed after a follow-up period of 9 months. Therefore, it is not recommended to stop treatment with IL-17 receptor antagonists even if there is complete clearance of psoriasis.

COMMENT

The article investigated the psoriasis recurrence in patients treated with brodalumab and when the treatment was stopped by Amgen in June 2015.

Patients were treated with brodalumab under Amgen's protocols and the drug development program was abruptly stopped. A retrospective multicenter cohort study was devised on these patients to see the relapse of psoriasis. The definition of relapse was request of the patient to start new treatment after stoppage of brodalumab.

Brodalumab is a recombinant human monoclonal antibody to the interleukin-

17A receptor. It is used in the treatment of moderate-to-severe plaque psoriasis. This decreases inflammatory pathways which are involved in immune mediated injury. Brodalumab is given in a dose of 210 mg subcutaneously at weeks 0, 1, 2 followed by every 2 weeks.

In this study 77 patients were followed up for a period of 9 months. All the 77 patients relapsed by 9 months. At the time of treatment stoppage 87% of patients had achieved PASI 90. The median time of relapse was 46 days with the duration ranging from 7 to 224 days. Total 73 patients relapsed with plaque psoriasis, 1 with erythrodermic psoriasis and 3 with pustular psoriasis. Only 7 patients who had no previous psoriatic arthritis relapsed with features of psoriatic arthritis.

Studies on relapse following treatment with other biologics also need to be done. If there is such a complete relapse following cessation of treatment with brodalumab, the cost factor should be considered while starting the patient on treatment since the patient would eventually need other systemic or topical agents on cessation of treatment or they should be able to continue treatment with biologics indefinitely.

Key Messages

- ***Sudden stoppage of treatment with brodalumab is associated with rapid relapse of psoriasis with some patients even presenting with more severe disease***
- ***Therefore, it is not advisable to stop treatment with brodalumab suddenly even in patients who have complete clearance of the disease since most of the patients in this study had achieved PASI 90 when the treatment was stopped***
- ***It is advisable to slowly taper the dose and simultaneously start the patient on other modes of treatment before complete cessation of therapy with brodalumab.***

ARTICLE 109

Emerging Targeted Therapies for Plaque Psoriasis – Impact of Ixekizumab

Kazemi T, Farahnik B, Koo J, et al. Emerging targeted therapies for plaque psoriasis - Impact of ixekizumab. ***Clin Cosmet Investig Dermatol. 2017;10:133-9.***

Abstract

The importance of interleukin 17 (IL-17) in psoriasis disease activity have provided a new target for biologic therapy. The US Food and Drug Administration (FDA) approved ixekizumab which seems to be a promising medication for psoriasis.

Results of phase III trials of ixekizumab have been reviewed to assess the efficacy and safety. The study also compared these results with other biologics like tildrakizumab and guselkumab, ustekinumab and brodalumab, and secukinumab.

The collective results from various studies demonstrate that ixekizumab achieves higher PASI 75 and similar or higher static Physician Global Assessment 0-1 rates than the other anti-IL-17 and anti-IL-23 agents.

Ixekizumab by exhibiting a vigorous clinical response with remarkable improvement in QoL found to be an extremely efficacious FDA-approved treatment for psoriasis.

COMMENT

Psoriasis is a chronic, relapsing immune-mediated inflammatory skin disorder. The plaque-type psoriasis (psoriasis vulgaris) is characterized by erythematous, well-circumscribed papules and plaques covered with silvery scales on extensor surfaces and other cutaneous locations.

Despite recent advancements, the immunopathogenesis of psoriasis remains incompletely understood. Basically, psoriasis is a T-helper (Th) 1 driven disease. Recently various studies have demonstrated a central role for Th17 cells in psoriasis, in disease etiology and treatment. Activated Th17 cells promote keratinocyte hyperproliferation through production and release of specific cytokines like IL-17 activates receptors on epithelial cells, B and T lymphocytes, fibroblasts, monocyte, and bone marrow.

This article is based on a comprehensive literature search using the PubMed database to identify published results of English language phase II and III clinical trials on IL-17 and IL-23 axis biologic agents, primarily ixekizumab, in order to report the percentage of psoriasis patients with a positive response to these agents.

Interleukin-23 and IL-17 are central in the pathogenesis of plaque psoriasis. Novel biologic agents are targeted against them. Anti-IL-17 biologics are brodalumab, secukinumab and ixekizumab. Brodalumab has been withdrawn from the market because of suicidal tendency of the drug.

Secukinumab is fully human anti-IL-17 IgG monoclonal antibody that is FDA approved for the treatment of moderate-to-severe plaque psoriasis. Among the four phase III trials comparing secukinumab 300 mg to placebo, the pooled proportion of patients achieving PASI 75 was more than 80% and Investigator Global Assessment 0–1 was 70% at 12 weeks.

Ixekizumab is a humanized monoclonal antibody that binds to and inhibits the IL-17 cytokine family. It is the most recently FDA-approved biologic treatment for moderate-to-severe plaque psoriasis. Three major phase III trials, UNCOVER-1, UNCOVER-2 and UNCOVER-3, were conducted to evaluate the efficacy, safety, and impact on quality of life of this new agent.

Though head to head trials are lacking, collective results from multiple studies showed ixekizumab achieves higher PASI 75 and static Physician Global Assessment (sPGA) 0-1 rates than other IL-17 inhibitors. Mild and moderate *candida* infections were more common in patients treated with ixekizumab, secukinumab, and brodalumab. Neutropenia was most commonly reported in patients treated with ixekizumab.

Ixekizumab at the most efficacious dosing (Q2W), achieves the highest PASI 75 of all IL-17 and IL-23 axis agents. More total injections are the notable disadvantage of ixekizumab. Phase III data reveal that among etanercept and other biologics such as secukinumab, brodalumab, tildrakizumab, guselkumab, and ustekinumab, ixekizumab achieves similar to superior results with a positive safety profile.

Key Messages

- *Ixekizumab is an extremely efficacious, newly FDA-approved treatment for moderate-to-severe plaque psoriasis that demonstrates a vigorous clinical response and significant improvement in patient quality of life*
- *Ixekizumab at the most efficacious dosing (Q2W) attains the highest PASI 75 of all IL-17 and IL-23 axis agents.*

ARTICLE 110

Infections from Seven Clinical Trials of Ixekizumab, an Anti-interleukin-17A Monoclonal Antibody, in Patients with Moderate-to-Severe Psoriasis

Papp KA, Bachelez H, Blauvelt A, et al. Infections from seven clinical trials of ixekizumab, an anti-interleukin-17A monoclonal antibody, in patients with moderate-to-severe psoriasis.
Br J Dermatol. 2017; 177(6):1537-51.

Abstract

It is common to note infections in psoriatic patients treated with biological therapies. The study outline the incidence of infections in psoriatic patients treated with ixekizumab. The data are summarized from an integrated database of seven controlled and uncontrolled ixekizumab psoriasis trials. The information is presented from patients exposed to ixekizumab, collected from all seven trials. UNCOVER-2 and UNCOVER-3 study compared ixekizumab with etanercept during the induction period. Incidence and exposure-adjusted incidence rates (IRs) per 100 patient-years (PYs) are reported.

The infections did not increase with long-term usage of ixekizumab. Among all patients treated with ixekizumab (all seven trials), the incidence of life threatening infections were low (2%, IR 1·3). Even candida infections, together with eight cases of esophageal candidiasis, were effectively managed with antifungal therapy and did not lead to discontinuation.

In general, infections occurred in a higher percentage of patients treated with ixekizumab vs. placebo during the first 12 weeks of treatment; however, specific infection rates were comparable largely across treatment groups. Incidences of grave infections were low and similar across treatment groups. The collective results from various studies demonstrate that ixekizumab achieves higher PASI 75 and similar or higher statistical Physician Global Assessment 0–1 rates than the other anti-IL-17 and anti-IL-23 agents.

Ixekizumab by exhibiting a vigorous clinical response with remarkable improvement in quality of life found to be an extremely efficacious FDA-approved treatment for psoriasis.

COMMENT

Biological therapies as such do not have any organ specific toxicity. But, it has side effects like infections, mainly mild upper respiratory tract infections.

UNCOVER-1, UNCOVER-2 and UNCOVER-3 are the trials in which the article has collected data regarding ixekizumab.

During the induction period for 12 weeks, 27% of ixekizumab group showed infections.

Upper respiratory tract and urinary tract infections are the most common infection reported. Cellulitis, appendicitis and erysipelas were very rarely reported. Infections are not related to period of exposure.

Totally only three patients had a recurrence of their previous serious infections. No active TB cases have been reported so far.

Candida infections were reported in quite high number. Oral candidiasis tops the list among fungal infection.

The set back of the study are lack of long-term comparisons. Comparison of ixekizumab to etanercept was only for 12 weeks and clinical trial populations are definitely not the representative of whole psoriasis population.

Key Messages

- *The infections seen in ixekizumab treated patients are Candida, staphylococcal and herpes zoster*
- *Infections overall did not increase with long-term ixekizumab exposure.*

ARTICLE 111

High Rate of Systemic Corticosteroid Prescription among Outpatient Visits for Psoriasis: A Population-based Epidemiological Study Using the Korean National Health Insurance Database

Eun SJ, Jang S, Lee JY, et al. High rate of systemic corticosteroid prescription among outpatient visits for psoriasis: A population-based epidemiological study using the Korean National Health Insurance database.
J Dermatol. 2017;44(9):1027-32.

Abstract

According to literature, systemic corticosteroids (SC) are not recommended for the treatment of psoriasis. Conversely many physicians often prescribe SC for patients with psoriasis. The study establishes the magnitude of SC prescription for outpatients with psoriasis in Korea. In regularity analysis for the full scale of prescribed SC, oral methylprednisolone was the most commonly prescribed SC, followed by dexamethasone and betamethasone injections. In multiple logistic regression analyses, the older age group and smaller healthcare institutions were more linked with the SC prescription. In conclusion, SC was usually prescribed for patients with psoriasis in Korea despite the current guidelines.

COMMENT

Inappropriate medications usage can have reflective medical consequences for elderly patients. It usually provides a large burden on the healthcare system.

According to literature, for psoriasis treatment systemic corticosteroids (SC) are not used. In clinical practice; however, many physicians frequently prescribe SC for patients with psoriasis for immediate results.

The article has used the 2010–2014 nationwide claims data of the Health Insurance Review and Assessment Service of Korea to verify the extent of SC prescription for outpatients with psoriasis in Korea and identify factors related with the use of SC.

The prevalence of improper prescribing remains alarmingly high for the elderly and particularly for nursing home residents. More studies are needed to document data regarding the adverse impact of improper prescribing on total healthcare costs and health outcomes of patients.

Mrowietz et al. states that literatures do not encourage systemic steroids in the treatment of psoriasis as the risk of disease deterioration was much higher after dose reduction or withdrawal. Contrarily, systemic steroids were the most commonly given drugs for psoriasis by general practitioners stated by German nationwide healthcare insurance.

There is no guideline-based evidence on systemic steroids causing rebound, erythroderma or pustular psoriasis.

To conclude, SC was broadly prescribed for psoriatic patients in Korea regardless of the current guidelines. Systemic corticosteroids use, greatly depends on institution characteristics and individuals. Since wide therapeutic options are available for psoriasis, use of steroids is controversy. More studies are required to assess the risk benefit ratio.

Key Messages

- ***Systemic corticosteroids were broadly prescribed for patients with psoriasis in Korea despite the current guidelines***
- ***More studies are required to assess the risk benefit ratio.***

ARTICLE 112

Hyperuricemia Is an Independent Risk Factor for Psoriatic Arthritis in Psoriatic Patients

Tsuruta N, Imafuku S, Narisawa Y. Hyperuricemia is an independent risk factor for psoriatic arthritis in psoriatic patients. *J Dermatol. 2017;44(12):1349-52.*

Abstract

Psoriatic arthritis (PsA) is mainly seen in psoriatic patients with plaques on the scalp, gluteal fold or nail lesions. The study establishes which psoriatic patients are prone to develop PsA.

Patients with and without PsA were statistically analyzed with respect to age, sex, age at onset, body mass index (BMI), smoking and drinking habits, familial history of psoriasis and comorbidities. Hyperuricemia is recognized to be more regular in psoriatic subjects than the normal population. Hyperuricemia may boost uric acid crystallization in and around joints, thereby inducing PsA in psoriatic subjects. Hyperuricemia appears to be a self-governing risk factor for PsA.

COMMENT

Psoriasis is a chronic inflammatory disease. Multiple types of psoriasis have been described, including pustular, guttate, and erythrodermic psoriasis, in addition to rarer forms such as psoriatic arthritis (PsA). It is often associated with features of the metabolic syndrome, including obesity, dyslipidemia, and type 2 diabetes. Psoriasis is also linked to an increased risk of incident cardiovascular disease (CVD). Hyperuricemia has been detected more frequently in patients with psoriasis and has also been associated with CVD. Specifically, the prevalence of CVD has been linked with higher levels of uric acid (UA). In addition, hyperuricemia has been reported to cause adverse cardiovascular outcomes, especially sudden cardiac death. In 1958, Walkerin first suggested that psoriasis may be associated with hyperuricemia.

Li Xin et al. describes that the correlation between psoriasis and hyperuricemia might be either ethnicity- or region-dependent. Kwon et al. recently proposed that an increased epidermal cell turnover could be an important cause of raised serum uric acid (SUA) levels among psoriatic patients.

Additional studies are required to determine the potential efficacy of systemic therapies for controlling SUA levels in psoriasis. Moreover, detection of increased SUAC levels in this patient population may enable earlier implementation of preventive measures for metabolic disturbances and awareness of CVD-associated risk of mortality.

Hyperuricemia in psoriatic patients could be simply a consequence of obesity and other coexisting metabolic disorders. Psoriasis itself might, at least in part, contribute directly to hyperuricemia, hence SUA levels should be routinely measured in psoriatic patients, and that the pharmacologic treatment of asymptomatic hyperuricemia might also be clinically relevant to the global treatment of patients.

Hyperuricemia is also known to be more frequent in psoriatic subjects than the normal population. Hyperuricemia may boost UA crystallization surrounding and in joints, thus inducing PsA in psoriatic subjects. Hyperuricemia appears to be an independent risk factor for PsA.

Key Messages

- ***Hyperuricemia is found to be more common in psoriatic subjects than the normal population***
- ***Hyperuricemia appears to be a self-governing risk factor for PsA.***

ARTICLE 113

How Is Disease Severity Associated with Quality of Life in Psoriasis Patients? Evidence from a Longitudinal Population-based Study in Sweden

Geale K, Henriksson M, Schmitt-Egenolf M. How is disease severity associated with quality of life in psoriasis patients? Evidence from a longitudinal population-based study in Sweden.
Health Qual Life Outcomes. 2017;15(1):151.

Abstract

The study was conducted to assess the impact of disease severity on generic quality of life (QoL) in psoriatic patients. The principle of this work was to investigate the relationship of psoriasis in life using a population-based dataset.

Severity was calculated by the Psoriasis Area and Severity Index (PASI). The generic EQ-5D-3L utility instrument, under the UK tariff, was used to compute QoL. The association between PASI and EQ-5D-3L was estimated using a Swedish psoriasis register (PsoReg).

The patient-level heterogeneity seems to be an important source of confounding when estimating the relationship between QoL and PASI.

The study shows that PASI appears to have a larger impact on QoL than previously estimated. Regular collection of generic QoL data in registers should be encouraged.

COMMENT

Psoriasis is manifested with erythematous papules or thickened plaques covered with silver-white scales. It causes daily life inconvenience like pruritus, burning sensation, dryness in the inflicted area. Negative influence on appearance like exfoliating epidermal residues, crumbled and pigmented fingernails is the biggest complaints.

Current treatment in standard medicine ranges from topical corticosteroid to human monoclonal antibody, immunosuppressants and phototherapy. While treatments in outpatient setting is quite enough for most patients, some patients having a sudden flare-up or in critical condition need to be hospitalized. Inpatient setting will offer more rigorous regimen of topical corticosteroid, systemic biological agents, or ultraviolet (UV) lights. The cost of management of psoriasis is often enormous due to life-long use of drugs and higher price from advanced therapy.

There are many ways to examine psoriasis severity. Psoriasis Area and Severity Index (PASI) is perceived as a gold standard. It uses standardized mathematic formula with each factors weighted to produce the total score by taking into account the body surface area (BSA) involvement, lesion location, the extent of redness and thickness.

Quality of life (QoL) is defined by World Health Organization as "the individuals' perception of their place in life, in the cultural and value systems in which they exist and in relation to their goals, expectations, standards and concerns." The description reveals the significance of subjective experience to QoL rather than healthcare worker's scrutiny.

The objective of this study was to demonstrate how register data can be utilized to provide longitudinal estimates of the connection between QoL and disease severity. The EuroQol- 5 Dimension (EQ-5D) is an instrument which evaluates the generic QoL developed in Europe and widely used. The five dimensions such as mobility, self-care, usual activities, pain/discomfort, and anxiety/depression are the EQ-5D descriptive system to measure health-related quality of life (HRQoL) with one question for each.

This study illustrates how register data can be used to derive the association between disease severity and QoL by exploiting the unique content and structure of registers.

Registers are a rich source of information, and this study has illustrated how they can be utilized if they include both disease severity and QoL. However, they can vary in both content and quality, and it is therefore important to evaluate the usefulness and representativeness of the data on a case-by-case basis with respect to the percentage of eligible patients, potential for bias, and which measures of severity and QoL are available. Routine collection of generic QoL data in registers should be encouraged to enable similar applications in other disease areas.

Key Messages

- ***Registers are a wealthy source of information, and this study has illustrated how they can be utilized if they include both disease severity and QoL***
- ***Regular collection of generic QoL data in registers should be encouraged.***

ARTICLE 114

Influence of TNF-alpha Inhibitors and Fumaric Acid Esters on Male Fertility in Psoriasis Patients

Heppt F, Colsman A, Maronna A, et al. Influence of TNF-alpha inhibitors and fumaric acid esters on male fertility in psoriasis patients.

J Eur Acad Dermatol Venereol. 2017;31(11):1860-6.

Abstract

This monocentric, open-label, prospective study is to find out any influence of a therapy with TNF-α inhibitors or fumaric acid esters on male fertility and sperm quality in patients with psoriasis.

The study collected semen samples from psoriatic patients receiving either TNF-α inhibitors or fumaric acid esters. Sperm parameters were assessed based on WHO definitions.

About 101 semen specimens from 27 patients were collected. At least one sperm/seminal abnormality is seen in 85.2% of patients. It also showed sperm parameters indicative of genital tract inflammation. No major gonadal dysfunction was observed in any patient.

The study documented genital tract inflammation as one of the vital comorbidity of psoriasis. The treatment with TNF-α inhibitors or fumaric acid esters has no major negative side effects on sperm quality.

COMMENT

This article throws light on the influence of Tumor necrosis factor (TNF)-α inhibitors and fumaric acid esters (FAE) on male fertility in psoriasis patients.

Tumor necrosis factor-α inhibitors like adalimumab, infliximab and etanercept are permitted for the treatment of moderate-to-severe chronic plaque psoriasis in adult patients who did not respond or contraindicated , or not tolerant to, other systemic therapies such as cyclosporine, methotrexate or psoralen and ultraviolet A (PUVA). The most common infections include lower respiratory tract and skin infections. Tuberculosis was shown to be the most common opportunistic infection.

Fumaric acid esters are chemical compounds derived from the unsaturated dicarbonic acid and fumaric acid. Fumaric acid esters have been proven to be an effective therapy in patients with psoriasis even though the mechanisms of action are not completely understood. The most common side effects are gastrointestinal symptoms such as abdominal pain, diarrhea, nausea and malaise. Less commonly observed side effects are lymphocytopenia, leukocytopenia and elevated eosinophil counts.

This article conducts a monocentric, open-label, prospective study in which semen analysis of patients taking TNF inhibitors and FAE. Complete analysis of semen based on WHO criteria was done at the beginning and repeated every 3 months.

More than 80% shows at least variations in one parameter. Azoospermia recorded in two patients. Nearly 50% shows inflammation of genital tract. No notable negative effects on sperm quality or mobility seen in FAE or TNF-α inhibitors.

Significant dysfunction of gonads is not noted in any patient. Along with other comorbidities of psoriasis, genital tract inflammation is added to the list.

Quality of sperm is not majorly affected on treatment with FAE or TNF-α inhibitors. However the study sample is only 27, further studies can be conducted with more patients.

Key Messages

- *Therapy with TNF-a inhibitors or fumaric acid esters did not have any harmful effects on relevant sperm parameters*
- *No major gonadal dysfunction was recorded in any patient.*

ARTICLE 115

Interval between Onset of Psoriasis and Psoriatic Arthritis Comparing the UK Clinical Practice Research Datalink with a Hospital-based Cohort

Tillett W, Charlton R, Nightingale A, et al. Interval between onset of psoriasis and psoriatic arthritis comparing the UK Clinical Practice Research Data link with a hospital-based cohort.
Rheumatology (Oxford). 2017;56(12):2109-13.

Abstract

The large, well-classified secondary care cohort study was conducted to demonstrate the time interval between the commencement of psoriasis and PsA in the UK primary care setting. Patients with PsA and/or psoriasis in the UK Clinical Practice Research Data link (CPRD) are included in the study. Comparisons were done with the time interval between diagnoses in the Bath cohort.

In both cohorts, the greater part of patients had psoriasis before their PsA diagnosis or within the same calendar year with only a marginal receiving their PsA diagnosis first (7.1 and 14.8%). The median time between psoriasis and PsA was 8 years in the CPRD and 7 years in the Bath cohort.

COMMENT

Psoriasis is a chronic skin disorder, now documented as one of the most common immune-mediated diseases. The severity of psoriasis can range from a mild disease involving small body surface area to extensive skin involvement and, in many cases, has a major impact on people's quality of life.

Psoriatic patients are at an increased risk for getting psoriatic arthritis (PsA) in their lifetime. Despite treatment advances with newly developed immune modulating agents such as tumor necrosis factor-α (TNF-α) inhibitors, patients with PsA still experience significant morbidity, including progressive joint destruction, functional disability, and increased healthcare costs. Therefore, early diagnosis and treatment of PsA is recommended to avoid disease-associated disability and loss of work place productivity. One of the major conundrums in the epidemiology of psoriasis and PsA is the prevalence of PsA in psoriasis patients.

So far no study has find out the true incidence and risk factors for PsA. The limitations are small studies, discriminating study populations, inadequate follow-up, and PsA classification criteria lacking diagnostic sensitivity.

This article finds out the interval between psoriasis and PsA. Patients with PsA and/or psoriasis, in the UK Clinical Practice Research Data link (CPRD) were considered in the study. The PsA longitudinal observational cohort study was taken as secondary care cohort. Both cohorts find that the greater part of patients had psoriasis before their PsA diagnosis or within the same year with only a marginal receiving their PsA diagnosis first.

Eight years is the median time between diagnoses in the CPRD and 7 years in the Bath cohort. Although, various studies have examined the risk factors for the development and progression of PsA, none have explored the psoriasis-specific disease features associated with an increased risk of PsA. The proinflammatory cytokine TNF-α has been shown to be expressed in the synovium, synovial lining, and skin lesions of PsA patients; therefore, it is plausible that larger psoriatic lesions may result in increased systemic levels of TNF-α and therefore play a role in PsA development.

All psoriasis patients should be screened for inflammatory arthritis to find the exact incidence of PsA in psoriasis.

Key Messages

- *It is mandatory to screen all psoriatic patients for psoriatic arthritis, since PsA experience significant morbidity, including progressive joint destruction, functional disability, and increased healthcare costs*
- *The median time between psoriasis and PsA diagnoses was 8 years in the CPRD and 7 years in the Bath cohort.*

ARTICLE 116

Increased Prevalence of HCV and Hepatic Decompensation in Adults with Psoriasis: A Population-based Study in the United Kingdom

Noe MH, Grewal SK, Shin DB, et al. Increased prevalence of HCV and hepatic decompensation in adults with psoriasis: A population-based study in the United Kingdom.
J Eur Acad Dermatol Venereol. 2017;31(10):1674-80.

Abstract

The population-based study in the United Kingdom is to find the association between the hepatitis C virus (HCV) and psoriasis.

To illustrate the prevalence of HCV in psoriasis patients compared to controls, and to find the incidence of hepatic decompensation in HCV+ psoriasis patients compared to HCV+ controls.
In fully adjusted models, a statistically noteworthy increase in prevalence was seen in the adults with psoriasis. Non-statistically considerable increased incidence of hepatic decompensation is seen in HCV+ patients with psoriasis than HCV+ individuals without psoriasis. Higher prevalence of HCV in adults with psoriasis and a higher rate of hepatic decompensation are noted.

COMMENT

Hepatitis C virus (HCV) related morbidity and mortality places a substantial burden on healthcare systems worldwide. This article find out the prevalence of HCV in psoriasis patients, compared to controls, and to the incidence of hepatic decompensation in HCV+ psoriasis patients compared to HCV+ controls.

After acute HCV infection occurs, 15% to 25% of subjects spontaneously clear viremia while 75% to 85% of individuals develop chronic HCV infection. Hepatitis C virus antibodies, HCV RNA elevated aminotransferase or histology detects the diagnosis. However, from 10% to 20% of subjects develop cirrhosis, generally in a time gap from 20 to 30 years.

Only few studies have evaluated the prevalence of the above-cited infectious disease in the psoriasis (PsO) population. In 2011, Yang et al. reported an increased prevalence of Hepatitis B virus (HBV) and HCV in PsO

Taiwanese patients. In 2010, Cohen et al. in their study performed in Israel found an increased prevalence of HCV but not of HBV in PsO compared to control. The different frequency of HBV and HCV infection, as well as of PsO worldwide, can account for the discrepancies among the data published so far.

Non-statistically considerable increased incidence of hepatic decompensation seen in HCV+ patients with psoriasis than HCV+ individuals without psoriasis.

This study results demonstrate a higher prevalence of HCV in adults with psoriasis and a higher rate of hepatic decompensation in HCV+ individuals with moderate-severe psoriasis.

It is essential that the HCV+ psoriasis patients should be referred to a hepatologist for expert clinical management.

Key Messages

- ***Hepatitis C virus (HCV) connected morbidity and mortality places a substantial burden on healthcare systems worldwide***
- ***This study results reveal a higher prevalence of HCV in adults with psoriasis and a higher rate of hepatic decompensation in HCV+ individuals with moderate-severe psoriasis.***

ARTICLE 117

Evaluation of Adherence Predictors for the Treatment of Moderate to Severe Psoriasis with Biologics: The Importance of Physician-patient Interaction and Communication

Zschocke I, Ortland C, Reich K. Evaluation of adherence predictors for the treatment of moderate to severe psoriasis with biologics: The importance of physician-patient interaction and communication.
J Eur Acad Dermatol Venereol. 2017;31(6):1014-20.

Abstract

The non-interventional retrospective study was conducted to analyze the treatment efficacy and adherence of biologic agents in moderate-to-severe psoriasis. Study data were analyzed for possible predictors of adherence in an explorative manner.

Based on the physician's assessment subsets of adherent and non-adherent patients were classified. The factors that were responsible for adherence are knowledge about comorbidities and previous treatment failure. Physician-patient communication seems to play a vital role in treatment and adherence part. Treating physicians should be attentive about soft aspects of interaction with the patient that might power treatment adherence.

COMMENT

Psoriasis is often perceived by patients as being incomprehensible, incurable and uncontrollable disease. It is the duty of dermatologists to convey to patients that the disease can generally be controlled, and provide hope that effective therapies are available.

This original article is a study conducted in Germany which includes Dermatologist and psoriatic patients. The study aims at finding out the evaluation of adherence predictors for the treatment of moderate-to-severe psoriasis with biologics and the importance of physician-patient interaction and communication.

The expectations differ from individual patients and treating physicians. The quality of life is severely affected in psoriatic patients.

Among various treatment options, biologics has placed a role in treating psoriatic patients. Biologics fulfil the patient satisfaction as well as disease control. Biologics has increased the patient expectations.

Compared to other treatments, biologics top the list in treatment satisfaction. A study conducted in Italy stated that adherence to treatment is directly proportional to patient doctor relationship.

Many biologics are available in the market, the choice depends on patient expectations. Psoriatic comorbidities and previous treatment failures play a vital role in current treatment adherence. Treatment adherence also influenced by patient-doctor interaction.

Psoriasis treatment guidelines should also recognize the importance of tailoring treatment to the needs of the individual patient.

Key Messages

- *Two main factors were identified on the patients' side that were positively linked to adherence: a lack of efficacy of the previous treatments and the knowledge of comorbidities associated with severe psoriasis*
- *Psoriasis treatment guidelines should also identify the significance of tailoring treatment to the needs of the individual patient.*

ARTICLE 118

Exploration of Candidate Biomarkers for Human Psoriasis Based on Gas Chromatography-mass Spectrometry Serum Metabolomics

Kang H, Li X, Zhou Q, et al. Exploration of candidate biomarkers for human psoriasis based on gas chromatography-mass spectrometry serum metabolomics.
Br J Dermatol. 2017;176(3):713-22.

Abstract

The study explore candidate biomarkers for human psoriasis based on gas chromatography-mass spectrometry serum metabolomics. The metabolome is the end products of proteomics or cellular processes that may be closely linked with the pathogenesis of psoriasis.

The study determines the differences in serum metabolomic profiles between psoriatic patients and healthy controls.

Compared with healthy controls, psoriatic patients had increased levels of amino acids such as asparagine, aspartic acid, isoleucine, phenylalanine, ornithine and proline; higher levels of lactic acid and urea; and lesser levels of crotonic acid, azelaic acid, ethanolamine and cholesterol.

The study found out that the glycolysis pathway and amino acid metabolic activity are amplified in patients with psoriasis. These metabolic perturbations are responsible for protein biosynthesis and keratinocyte hyperproliferation. The metabolomics involved in the pathogenesis of psoriasis and provide insights into early diagnosis and therapeutic intervention.

COMMENT

Psoriasis is a chronic inflammatory disease affecting up to 3% of the world's population. Histologically, psoriasis is characterized by hyper proliferative keratinocytes and infiltration of prominent T cells, dendritic cells and neutrophils in the dermis. Despite multiple studies, the etiology and immunopathogenesis of psoriasis have not been fully understood. In addition, identifying biomarkers for psoriasis diagnosis and treatment response is still a daunting task in the field due to the heterogeneity of disease.

This article by Kang et al. using a systems metabolomics approach provides candidate biomarkers. The end products of proteomics are metabolome and that may be closely associated with the pathogenesis of psoriasis.

Multiple studies have analyzed metabolomics which are by product in various pathways. Metabolites are different in pre and post treatment and it reflects Psoriasis Area Severity Index (PASI), hence these metabolites can be considered as marker to assess disease severity. Mass spectrometry such as gas chromatography or liquid chromatography can be used. Gas chromatography is considerably of less cost.

Compared with healthy controls, psoriatic patients had increased levels of amino acids such as asparagine, aspartic acid, isoleucine, phenylalanine, ornithine and proline; very high levels of lactic acid and urea; and lesser levels of crotonic acid, azelaic acid, ethanolamine and cholesterol.

Psoriatic patients had increased glycolysis pathway. Lactic acid levels in psoriatic patients are more compared to their controls. In the complex pathogenesis of psoriasis, metabolites also play a role. Metabolites can be used as a tool to diagnose and assess severity.

Key Messages

- ***Psoriasis had increased levels of amino acids such as asparagine, aspartic acid, isoleucine, phenylalanine, ornithine and proline; higher amounts of lactic acid and urea; and lesser levels of crotonic acid, azelaic acid, ethanolamine and cholesterol***
- ***More works are warranted to further validate these metabolic biomarkers.***

ARTICLE 119

Increased Frequencies of Basophils, Type 2 Innate Lymphoid Cells and Th2 Cells in Skin of Patients with Atopic Dermatitis but not Psoriasis

Mashiko S, Mehta H, Bissonnette R, et al. Increased frequencies of basophils, type 2 innate lymphoid cells and Th2 cells in skin of patients with atopic dermatitis but not psoriasis.
J Dermatol Sci. 2017;88(2):167-74.

Abstract

Atopic dermatitis (AD) has been considered to be primarily Th2 mediated. Basophils, innate lymphoid cells type 2, Th2 cells and mast cells are type 2 cells. Atopic dermatitis patients also have high levels of IL-13 and IL-4. The presence and interaction of type 2 cells and IL-4 and 13 source in the serum and cutis of patients with psoriasis and AD were analyzed. Flow cytometry was used to analyze interleukin levels. There was more significant elevation of Th2, basophils and ILC2 but not mast cells in skin of atopic dermatitis patients compared to psoriasis patients. This elevation was not seen in serum levels. More interleukin expression especially 4 and 13 was seen in cutaneous T cells of AD patients compared to psoriasis. All this indicates the use of targeting IL-13 and 4 signaling pathways in patients with AD.

COMMENT

Asthma and atopic dermatitis (AD) have innate lymphoid cells in inflammation process. Inflammatory cytokines are released. Cutis of AD individuals has higher proportion of interleukin C2s. Prostaglandin D2, interleukins like 33 and 25 and thymic stromal lymphopoietin are more evident in AD cutis.

Atopic dermatitis cutis also shows increased basophils. Elimination of IL-4 production results in reduced inflammatory response. Natural cytotoxicity receptor on stimulation with interleukins 13 and 4 up regulates the keratinocytes.

Interleukin 22 is responsible for the skin thickening in psoriatic disease. IL-17F and IL-17A leads to the inflammation by neutrophils.

Atopic dermatitis patient's innate lymphoid cells manufacture array of interleukins like 13, 5, 6 and 4. After allergen contact, type 2 cytokines are produced in large number, which is evident in patient gut, blood, respiratory organ and skin.

Key Message

- *The study has found out that the occurrence of group 2 innate lymphoid cells is elevated in cutis of AD patients compared to controls.*

ARTICLE 120

Initiation, Switching, and Cessation of Psoriasis Treatments among Patients with Moderate to Severe Psoriasis in the United States

Armstrong AW, Koning JW, Rowse S, et al. Initiation, switching, and cessation of psoriasis treatments among patients with moderate to severe psoriasis in the United States.
Clin Drug Investig. 2017;37(5):493-501.

Abstract

This retrospective, longitudinal cohort study analyze initiation, switching, and cessation of psoriasis treatments among patients with moderate-to-severe psoriasis in the United States.

The study aimed to identify patterns of treatment transitions of US patients with moderate-to-severe psoriasis over 5 years. Under treatment of moderate-to-severe psoriasis found to be common.

COMMENT

Psoriatic treatment options are wide range for the past few decades starting from coal tar to current biologics. In spite of multiple therapies, 100% cure rate is not attainable in psoriasis, this lead to large dissatisfaction of patient. Naturally, patients switch among various treatment modalities. In the current trend, switching among therapies is acceptable to improve patient quality of life. To prevent high cumulative dose rotational therapy was also encouraged.

Patients are in search of a drug with good result with almost no side effects. Switching between therapies are seen to improve the standard of living among psoriatic patients.

The article deals with the retrospective, longitudinal cohort study in which US patients with psoriasis for 5 years. The study found out that a total of 81,000 of 346,000 patients had switched treatment in the preceding year. Under treatment of moderate-to-severe psoriasis appeared to be common.

Since switching among therapy is acceptable no clear cut guidelines regarding switching of therapies are available. More studies are needed to illustrate about switching of therapy. When present treatment is not effective, switching of therapy gives patient an option to move to other responsive therapy.

Key Messages

- ***Switching psoriasis treatment is a common, accepted practice that is used to improve disease management and improve patient outcomes***
- ***Under treatment of moderate-to-severe psoriasis appeared to be common.***

ARTICLE 121

Limited Presence of IL-22 Binding Protein, a Natural IL-22 Inhibitor, Strengthens Psoriatic Skin Inflammation

Martin JC, Wolk K, Bériou G, et al. Limited presence of IL-22 binding protein, a natural IL-22 inhibitor, strengthens psoriatic skin inflammation.
J Immunol. 2017;198(9):3671-8.

Abstract

Psoriasis is a chronic inflammatory disease resulting from dysregulated immune activation associated with a large local secretion of cytokines. Interleukin (IL)-22 induces proinflammatory chemokines and antimicrobial peptides and inhibits the terminal differentiation of keratinocytes thereby contribute to inflammation and epithelial remodeling of the psoriatic skin. The action of IL-22 is regulated by IL-22 binding protein (IL-22BP). The strong IL-22 increase in lesional psoriatic skin was associated with a moderate induction of IL-22BP. The study found positive correlations with the expression of IL-22-inducible molecules (IL-20, IL-24, IL-36γ, CXCL1, and BD2) in keratinocytes. Finally, psoriasis severity was strongly correlated with serum IL-22/IL-22BP protein ratio. The study proposes that though IL-22BP can control deleterious actions of IL-22 in the skin, its limited production prevents an adequate neutralization of IL-22 and contributes to the development and maintenance of epidermal alterations in psoriasis.

COMMENT

Psoriasis is a chronic inflammatory skin disease that affects approximately 2% of the Caucasian population. It is generally acknowledged that skin changes result from chronic dysregulated activation of the cutaneous immune system that is by secreted cytokines which alters the biology of local tissue cells.

In large quantities IL-22 is present in psoriatic lesions. CD4+ T cell populations and group 3 innate lymphoid cells are main producers of IL-22. Because the expression of the membrane IL-22R is restricted to epithelial/epithelioid cells, IL-22 assumes major cross-talk functions between immune and epithelial cells, especially at body barriers. IL-22 induces proinflammatory chemokines and antimicrobial peptides and inhibits the terminal differentiation of keratinocytes thereby contribute to inflammation and epithelial remodeling of the psoriatic skin. Interestingly, the IL-22 activity is regulated by IL-22 binding protein (IL-22BP). IL-22 binding protein is a soluble single chain receptor encoded by the gene *IL22RA2* that particularly prevents the binding of IL-22 to IL-22R.

Psoriasis-like skin inflammation was induced in the right ear of *Il22ra2+/+* and *Il22ra2–/–* rats, and in the back skin of C57BL/6J mice as previously described. Briefly, topical application of Aldara cream (3M Pharmaceuticals) was performed daily for 5 days. Skin thickness was measured daily with a Digimatic caliper and the percentage of skin thickness increase relative to day 0 was calculated every day. Animals were sacrificed at day 5 for qRT-PCR and histopathological analyses were done on skin tissues. Skin sections were stained with H&E.

The study found out that psoriatic skin shows relative IL-22BP deficiency. IL-22BP deficiency exacerbates imiquimod-induced skin inflammation in the rat. IL-22BP blockade exacerbates imiquimod-induced skin inflammation in the mouse. IL-22/IL-22BP ratio correlates with the expression of IL-22 target molecules in psoriasis. IL-22 induces IL-24 expression in keratinocytes. Ratio of IL-22 and IL-22BP blood protein levels correlates with psoriasis disease severity.

The study showed that IL-22BP critically controls deleterious actions of IL-22 during skin inflammation in rodents and suggest it is insufficiently present to limit the extent of IL-22 pathogenicity in human psoriasis.

Key Messages

- *Psoriatic skin shows relative IL-22BP deficiency*
- *The serum IL-22/IL-22BP protein ratio strongly correlated with psoriasis severity.*

ARTICLE 122

Long-term Safety and Effectiveness of Adalimumab for Moderate to Severe Psoriasis: Results from 7-year Interim Analysis of the ESPRIT Registry

Menter A, Thaçi D, Wu JJ, et al. Long-term safety and effectiveness of adalimumab for moderate to severe psoriasis: Results from 7-year interim analysis of the ESPRIT Registry.
Dermatol Ther (Heidelb). 2017;7(3):365-81.

Abstract

Based on 7-year ESPRIT registry, the article assesses the long-term safety, effectiveness, and patient-reported outcomes (PROs) of adalimumab. Life-threatening and minor adverse effects are assessed. Deaths due to emerging adverse reactions are very less. Overall, adalimumab has a positive safety profile. The effectiveness of adalimumab was maintained for 7 years according to registry.

COMMENT

Psoriasis has multiple treatment options. Biologics are used extensively in psoriasis treatment in this decade. Tumor necrosis factor (TNF)-α has a major role in psoriatic complex pathogenesis. Tumor necrosis factor-α inhibitors are infliximab, adalimumab (ADA) and etanercept. The journal assesses the overall effectiveness and safety of ADA.

The data are used from a psoriatic register. The register was maintained for 7 years. Effectiveness is monitored based on physician global assessment. The study notes the life-threatening and minor adverse effects.

Less than 1 % patients had serious emergencies of cardiovascular and malignancy.

The main limitation of the article is it does not have controls.

No new threats to ADA were detected. Reported deaths to ADA were very minimal. The study goes in hand with other studies in safety terms. Overall, positive safety profile is given to ADA. This positive safety profile continues for 7 years.

Key Messages

- ***In this 7-year interim analysis, no new safety signals were observed and safety was steady with the known safety profile of ADA***
- ***The number of treatment-emergent deaths in the registry was below the expected rate for comparable general population.***

ARTICLE 123

Lymphopenia and CD4+/CD8+ Cell Reduction under Fumaric Acid Esters

Sondermann W, Rompoti N, Leister L, et al. Lymphopenia and CD4+/CD8+ cell reduction under fumaric acid esters. *Dermatology. 2017;233(4):295-302.*

Abstract

Psoriatic patients are treated with fumaric acid esters (FAEs). During psoriasis therapy, this cohort examine the control of FAEs on leukocytes, lymphocytes, and CD4+ and CD8+ cells. The study analyzes the T cell subsets.

The median lymphocyte count was appreciably reduced after the first 6 months of FAE therapy. About 11% showed severe lymphopenia. Significant reduction of CD4+ and CD8+ cell counts were observed.

The study warrants episodic monitoring of absolute lymphocyte counts and determination of T cell subsets before and during FAE therapy.

COMMENT

Psoriasis is a chronic skin disease associated with increased morbidity and mortality. Efficient and safe long-term treatment options are required to manage the illness successfully. A number of systemic agents are available; however, each of them has its own significant side effects.

Fumaric acid esters (FAEs) derivative of unsaturated dicarbonic acid fumaric acid used as monotherapy in psoriasis; supported by multiple studies in German. The most common side effects during induction therapy are flushing and gastrointestinal side effects such as nausea, vomiting and diarrhea which may lead to treatment discontinuation in as many as 30% of the patients. Leukopenia (particularly lymphopenia) is a concern during long-term FAE treatment. A decrease of lymphocytes below 500/mm^3 should lead to dosage reduction or withdrawal of treatment.

Various studies in psoriasis have already shown peripheral blood lymphopenia during oral FAE therapy. Smaller studies also documented a reduction of CD4+ and CD8+ cell counts. The article assesses the CD4+ and CD8+ cells and lymphocyte levels after FAE therapy. One-third of FAE treated patient had decreased white blood cells. Reduced lymphocyte levels are noted in more than half of treated patients.

CD8+ cells are very much reduced compared to CD4+ cells. The ratios of CD4+/CD8+ are increased in FAE treated patients.

Progressive multifocal leukoencephalopathy is the opportunistic infection noted in FAE treated patients. Reduced lymphocyte levels remain for lifelong as a scar.

Level of white blood cells and CD4 and CD 8 should be recorded before and after therapy.

Key Messages

- *Even after stopping FAE lymphopenia resembles a "hematological scar"*
- *Periodic monitoring of lymphocyte count is mandatory for patients treated with FAE.*

ARTICLE 124

Magnetic Resonance Imaging in Psoriatic Arthritis: A Descriptive Study of Indications, Features and Effect on Treatment Change

Maldonado-Ficco H, Sheane BJ, Thavaneswaran A, et al. Magnetic resonance imaging in psoriatic arthritis: A descriptive study of indications, features and effect on treatment change.
J Clin Rheumatol. 2017;23(5):243-5.

Abstract

The indications and features of axial/peripheral joint magnetic resonance imaging (MRI) in psoriatic arthritis (PsA) are evaluated in this study.

The study gathered scan details from the radiologist's official report. The major indications for MRI were for inflammatory or degenerative disease. Sacroiliac joint involvement is the most common involvement. About 70% of psoriatic patients had inflammatory arthritis in MRI diagnosis. In more than 50% MRI findings influenced treatment change.

Magnetic resonance imaging can be used as an addition to clinical examination in determining treatment change in some cases.

COMMENT

Psoriatic arthritis (PsA) can be diagnosed clinically, skiagram and magnetic resonance imaging (MRI). The study evaluates the indications and features of axial/peripheral joint MRI in PsA.

Magnetic resonance imaging helps in finding the exact location of inflammation which is not possible by clinical examination. Magnetic resonance imaging scan records were pooled from multiple scan centers. Inflammatory and degenerative diseases are the two main indicators for MRI. Sacroiliac joint involvement tops the list.

Fifty years was found to be the mean age. Slight female preponderance was noted. Mean duration of PsA was almost 11 years. Magnetic resonance imaging findings influenced treatment change more than half of the patients.

Magnetic resonance imaging helps in catching the early inflammation of joints. Treatment can be started before significant damage if PsA detected early by MRI.

Skiagram detects only at a later stage. When there is a clinical dilemma MRI is mandatory to detect and start earlier treatment for PsA.

Key Message

- *Magnetic resonance imaging is useful in evaluating patients with active PsA, particularly when suspecting inflammation and radiographic findings are unhelpful.*

ARTICLE 125

Minimal Disease Activity in Patients with Psoriatic Arthritis Treated with Ustekinumab: Results from a 24-week Real-world Study

Napolitano M, Costa L, Caso F, et al. Minimal disease activity in patients with psoriatic arthritis treated with ustekinumab: Results from a 24-week real-world study.
Clin Rheumatol. 2017;36(7):1589-93.

Abstract

Forty percent of psoriatic patients have psoriatic arthritis (PsA). This study researched treatment with ustekinumab (UST) in the context of a real-world setting. The study enrolled 34 PsA patients who had conventional treatment failure. Minimum disease activity was achieved by 70% at week 24. A sub-analysis also showed significant improvement in Psoriasis Area Severity Index score. The efficacy and safety of UST in PsA is assessed by the achievement of MDA, significant improvement in DLQI and nil adverse events in the context of a real-life setting.

COMMENT

Psoriatic arthritis (PsA) has features like synovitis, axial disease, enthesitis or dactylitis and psoriasis. According to Proton Rahman et al., PsA also affects up to 30–40% of patients with psoriasis. Multiple studies from the last two decades have shown that PsA is frequently an erosive and deforming disease in 40–60% of patients if diagnosed within the first few years.

Psoriatic arthritis has been associated with impaired physical function, reduced quality of life (QoL) and increased mortality, with about 20% of patients eventually developing a highly destructive and disabling form of PsA. Manifestations of PsA contribute to disease burden due to the negative effects on the patient's psychological and psychosocial functioning, dissatisfaction with the management of the disease and the negative impact on daily living activities.

The study uses minimal disease activity (MDA) criteria to identify a state of low disease activity, one of the principal goals of treatment for psoriatic disease. This study investigated treatment with ustekinumab (UST) in the context of a real-world setting.

The study observed at 24 weeks more than two-third of study population has achieved MDA. A sub-analysis of dermatological indices of the MDA criteria showed that the Psoriasis Area Severity Index score was considerably improved and body surface area was appreciably decreased at 24 weeks compared with that at baseline. The rheumatological indices also show remarkable improvement with UST at 24 weeks.

The study based on dermatological and rheumatological indices improvement confirms the efficacy and safety of UST in PsA. The study sample size is quite less. Further studies are needed with larger population.

Key Message

- *The study based on dermatological and rheumatological indices improvement confirms the efficacy and safety of ustekinumab in PsA.*

ARTICLE 126

Evidence and Suggested Therapeutic Approach in Psoriasis of Difficult-to-Treat Areas: Palmoplantar Psoriasis, Nail Psoriasis, Scalp Psoriasis, and Intertriginous Psoriasis

Sarma N. Evidence and suggested therapeutic approach in psoriasis of difficult-to-treat areas: Palmoplantar psoriasis, nail psoriasis, scalp psoriasis, and intertriginous psoriasis.
Indian J Dermatol. 2017;62(2):113-22.

Abstract

The management of a case of psoriasis is challenging as the disease is known for its chronic relapsing nature. The treatment options range from topical forms for milder disease and systemic drugs in case of severe disease. Also, the disease is proven to be associated with psychiatric ailments like depression, anxiety and suicidal tendencies. This article provides the treatment options for difficult-to-treat locations by compiling the review articles featuring the treatment guidelines for difficult-to-treat locations. The level of evidence presented in this article is based on Oxford center for evidence based medicine 2011.

COMMENT

This article focusses on the treatment of psoriasis on the difficult-to-treat areas like the scalp, nails, intertriginous areas and palmoplantar psoriasis. The treatment options for any conditions are based on evidence-based approach these days and the treatment for psoriasis is no exception. The article has been prepared after reviewing articles on management of psoriasis and treatment options are listed based on the level of evidence based upon Oxford centre for evidence based medicine 2011.

The management of palmoplantar psoriasis is difficult as the presentation of this condition overlaps with chronic eczema. Treatment of this variant of psoriasis is challenging as this is associated with pain and decrease in the quality of life. The topical treatment is the first-line of management for this condition. Emollients are to be considered as the first-line of treatment in this condition and has to be added as an adjuvant with other topical agents. Though topical high potent corticosteroids are efficacious, they could not be used for long-term (>12 weeks) in view of their side effect profile.

The other topical agents found safe and usable for long-term treatment of palmoplantar psoriasis are topical tazarotene, calcipotriol and PUVAsol/pPUVA (Paint PUVA). Topical coal tar in higher strengths are found to be effective and can be considered as second-line option. Excimer laser of 308 nm is safe and effective but costly treatment. Methotrexate is the drug considered as first choice when topical treatment fails. Acitretin can be used in cases where methotrexate fails. Apremilast and biologics like infliximab, secukinumab can be tried as third-line options.

Nail psoriasis has a significant impact on the quality of life and is often painful and is the most difficult to treat. Topical tazarotene, calcipotriol and anthralin are the first choice of topical agents. Topical corticosteroids preferably in lacquer formulation can be used in combination with other topical treatment to reduce the side effects. Intralesional triamcinolone acetonide can be used in isolated nail disease but the injection can be painful. Methotrexate and acitretin are the first-line systemic agents. Cyclosporine is used as a second-line systemic agent. Biologics though effective can be considered as third-line of treatment.

Scalp psoriasis presents with itchy lesions and response to the medications is poor. Topical treatment with corticosteroids are considered efficacious and first-line but preferably used for short duration. Topical calcipotriene is safe for long-term use but not efficacious as the sole therapy. Topical salicylic acid can be added for removing scales. Topical coal tar and dithranol can also be tried as they are cheap and quite effective. Systemic agents like methotrexate, cyclosporine and acitretin can be used when the above treatment fails.

Intertriginous psoriasis or inverse psoriasis frequently misdiagnosed as intertrigo is challenging to treat as high potent steroids cannot be used because of the location and irritation associated with other agents. Topical calcipotriol is considered as the first-line agent and can be used for long-term treatment. Topical mid-potent/mild steroids can be used initially when response to calcipotriol is minimal. Calcineurin inhibitors can also be tried and safe in long-term. Systemic agents can be tried when topical treatment fails.

Key Messages

- ***Evidence-based medicine is the most precise method of compiling the available scientific data***
- ***Many social, religious, economical, and regional factors are to be considered before proposing any therapeutic recommendation***
- ***This article provides updated evidence on the management of psoriasis of difficult-to-treat areas and suggests practical, scientific and logical treatment options for these conditions.***

ARTICLE 127

Topical Therapies for Psoriasis

Torsekar R, Gautam MM. Topical therapies in psoriasis.
Indian Dermatol Online J. 2017;8:235-45.

Abstract

The therapeutic ladder of psoriasis begins with topical therapy in mild cases and systemic therapy for moderate-to-severe disease. The commonly used topical therapy is topical corticosteroids which are most effective initially but cannot be used for a longer period because of their side effects. The other agents which can be used are topical calcipotriol which is safer when used in concentrations not exceeding 100 g per week. The other drugs like coal tar and anthralin can be used but side effects like messy application, smell and irritant contact dermatitis limits their use. The management of flexural psoriasis is still more difficult with application of milder drugs because of their location. Topical calcipotriol and tacrolimus can be used commonly for flexural psoriasis. Tazarotene can be used alone or in combination with topical steroids.

COMMENT

Topical therapies for psoriasis is indicated when the body surface involvement is <10%. If the involvement is more, then systemic treatment is given. Also, in areas like face and genitals, topical therapies can be tried. They can be given along with systemic treatment also.

The various factors determining the efficacy of topical therapies depend upon proper patient education, area of application, choice of vehicle, occlusion used and the combination method used.

Emollients and moisturizers are the backbone of psoriasis treatment as they are mainstay to decrease the dryness and scaling associated with the disease condition. The mechanism of action is regulating differentiation and apoptosis mechanism. They are also important in the sense that they help in the penetration of other topical agents. However, the drawback is that they cannot be used as monotherapy. In palmoplantar psoriasis, emollients play a major role in decreasing the need for other topical treatments and reducing pain and itching. They are available in various formulations like lotions, creams and soap substitutes. The side effects noted are folliculitis, allergic contact dermatitis and acne.

Anthralin is another topical agent which was widely used in the past. This drug has regained its use as a topical agent in the recent years because of its efficacy. The drug is used in cases of stable plaque psoriasis and is best avoided in areas like axilla and groins because of irritation. This drug probably has an anti-mitotic effect and thereby reduces keratinocyte proliferation. The commonly used concentration is 1% in lotion or cream formulation, initially used for 5 minutes and later the duration of treatment can be increased till irritation develops. Salicylic acid can also be used in combination to increase the penetration of dithranol. The side effects include irritant contact dermatitis and staining of clothes.

Coal tar was successfully used in few decades back as a part of Goeckerman regimen which was an inpatient procedure. The mechanism by which it acts are by inhibiting the DNA synthesis thereby reducing keratinocyte proliferation. The side effects noted are irritation, burning sensation, folliculitis and odor. It is available in the concentrations of 1% to 15%.

Salicylic acid is a topical keratolytic agent which is used in conjunction with other treatments to increase the penetration of other agents. The mechanism of action by inhibiting the cohesiveness between the keratinocytes and thereby causes shedding of scales. The combination with topical steroids can be used in areas of thick scales like the palms and soles. It is generally used in concentrations from 3-6% preferably in combination with a steroid or other topical agent. The side effects are irritation, burning sensation and symptoms of salicylism if applied for larger body surface areas. The symptoms of salicylism include tinnitus, nausea, vomiting, central nervous system symptoms and metabolic acidosis.

Calcineurin inhibitors like tacrolimus and pimecrolimus are used as off-label indication in psoriasis. These drugs act by inhibiting calcineurin thereby and also blocks the release of IL-2 and other cytokines. The concentration of tacrolimus available is 0.03–0.1% and the concentration of pimecrolimus is 1%. These drugs are not effective in treating chronic plaque psoriasis but can be used in flexural psoriasis. To increase the penetration, salicylic acid can be combined with it. The most common side effect reported is irritation and there is a theoretical risk of malignancy.

Tazarotene is a synthetic retinoid used in the topical treatment of psoriasis of the skin and nails. The formulations available for this drug are gel and cream in 0.1% and 0.05%. It can be used either alone or in combination with steroids and other topical agents. The mechanism of action is by binding to retinoic acid receptors and finally formation of gene response elements thereby affecting epidermal differentiation. Its side effects are irritation and photosensitivity. It is best avoided in the areas like face and intertriginous areas. It is contraindicated in pregnancy. Bexarotene 1% is a new retinoid effective in mild-to-moderate psoriasis.

Topical steroids are the most commonly used topical agents which can also be considered as the first-line treatment in psoriasis. The mechanism of action of steroids is vasoconstriction, immune modulatory and anti-inflammatory action. The classification for steroids ranges from mild potency to super potency steroids. However, the limitation of topical steroids is that it cannot be given for a longer period and the potency of steroids varies according to the body area used. It is classified as a pregnancy category C. Mild and moderate potent steroid are suitable for use in children instead of high potent steroids. Also, the formulation varies according to the areas of the body.

Vitamin D analogues are used in chronic plaque psoriasis as well as in flexural psoriasis and scalp psoriasis. The mechanism of action is by binding to vitamin D receptors and thereby changing regulates the epidermal differentiation. Calcipotriene is the commonly used analogue in concentration of 0.005%. It has similar efficacy as steroids with less side effects but as monotherapy it takes a longer time to produce response. The most common side effects associated with this drug is irritation, hypercalcemia if drug is used >100 g per week. The drug belongs to pregnancy category C.

Key Messages

- *Topical therapies are the first-line of treatment in mild cases of psoriasis*
- *Among topical therapies, topical steroids are the most commonly used, but for shorter duration*
- *New vehicle formulations like gels, creams, lotions, foams and shampoos are available.*

ARTICLE 128

Psoriasis and Comorbid Diseases: Implications for Management

Takeshita J, Grewal S, Langan SM, et al. Psoriasis and comorbid diseases: Implications for management. *J Am Acad Dermatol. 2017;76(3):393-403.*

Abstract

Psoriasis is a known risk factor for cardiovascular disease. This article implicates the association of psoriasis with other comorbidities including hepatic disease, chronic kidney disease, malignancies, infections, mood disorders and inflammatory bowel disease. Knowing and recognizing all this is necessary for proper care of psoriatic patients.

COMMENT

Cardiovascular risk factors are under-diagnosed and undertreated in cases of psoriasis. Methotrexate and tumor necrosis factor inhibitors (TNFi) have shown to reduce the incidence of cardiovascular events. Screening of patients with moderate-to-severe plaque psoriasis for cardiovascular risk factors should be carried out and moreover lifestyle modifications such as cessation of smoking and weight loss is to be advised to patients who are smokers and overweight. Loss of weight in obese individuals is known to help the Psoriasis Area Severity Index (PASI) score as well as it increases response to treatment.

Since psoriasis is also associated with hypertension, a blood pressure screening is recommended for psoriatic patients. This is also important before starting the patient on cyclosporine.

A screening for diabetes is also to be done in cases of psoriasis especially due to the increased risk of vascular complications and more aggressive diabetes in cases of psoriasis than in those without psoriasis. Patients of psoriasis also have increased prevalence of dyslipidemia indicating the necessity of a lipid screening test. Moreover, it is necessary for starting the patient on acitretin and cyclosporine.

There is also increased incidence of inflammatory bowel disease in cases of psoriasis. TNFi such as infliximab and adalimumab are useful for both treatment of psoriasis as well as ulcerative colitis and Crohn's disease. Methotrexate, acitretin and TNFi should be avoided in cases of psoriasis associated with liver disease.

There is increased incidence of psoriatic arthritis (PsA) especially with increased duration of the disease. Therefore, patients with psoriasis should be screened for PsA especially since systemic therapy is needed in cases of PsA.

There is increased incidence of mood disorders in cases of psoriasis. There is a common pathogenic mechanism apart from the chronic course of the disease leading to depression and anxiety. Since, acitretin and apremilast have known to cause mood disorders, these drugs are to be used with caution in patients prone to these disorders.

There is increased risk of melanoma and non-melanoma skin cancer (NMSC) in patients treated with TNFi. Psoralen and ultraviolet A (PUVA) therapy is also known to have increased risk of leading to NMSC. Patients on immunotherapy and phototherapy should be screened for the associated skin cancers annually.

Infections are commonly seen in patients treated with immunosuppressive agents. Therefore, appropriate vaccinations should be completed before the start of immunosuppressive agents. Screening for human immunodeficiency virus (HIV), Hepatitis B and C and tuberculosis should be done before inception of immunosuppressive therapies.

Key Messages

- *There are variety of disorders associated with psoriasis including hypertension, diabetes, obesity, cardiovascular events, inflammatory bowel disease, psoriatic arthritis, infections and malignancies*
- *Caution must be exerted while giving medication for the treatment of psoriasis and appropriate screening must be done according to the drug being given and the associated conditions.*

ARTICLE 129

Translating Psoriasis Guidelines into Practice: Important Gaps Revealed

Bhushan R, Lebwohl MG, Gottlieb AB, et al. Translating psoriasis guidelines into practice: Important gaps revealed. *J Am Acad Dermatol. 2016;74(3):544-51.*

Abstract

American Academy of Dermatology (AAD) devised certain educational sessions based on pre-existing guidelines for the treatment of psoriasis and psoriatic arthritis. The effectiveness of these guidelines in improvement of patient care was studied 6 months after the last session and 2.5 years after the first session by means of surveys. More than 92% of physicians reported improvement in knowledge with these sessions.

COMMENT

There are a set of published evidence-based clinical guidelines in the treatment of psoriasis and psoriatic arthritis. However, it is not being adhered to. This is not necessarily because of entrenched practices among physicians but might be because of lack of knowledge in implementing the guidelines. There are always newer advances in medicine and educational sessions that help physicians to keep abreast of the newer developments. All physicians may not be open to try out newer medications without proper evidence.

In this study, the effectiveness of these training sessions on the basis of guidelines were studied. Follow-up surveys were done after 6 months of the last session and after 2.5 years of the first session. Pre-session surveys were also conducted.

In both the follow-ups, 92% of subjects reported improvement in knowledge. This included improvement in assessment of comorbidities, severity, quality of life, counseling and confidence in treating patients with psoriasis and psoriatic arthritis. More than half of the subjects reported change in practice and more than 97% considered the sessions to potentially have a positive impact on their practice.

Self-reported data based on surveys, absence of controls and subject bias are limitations of this study.

An objective method of assessment of implementation of guidelines and also improvement in the severity of disease in the patients also need to be assessed.

Key Message

- ***The translating evidence into practice sessions created by the American Academy of Dermatology was useful and educative in the treatment of psoriasis and psoriatic arthritis as reported by physicians who undertook the sessions.***